Why Animals Don't Get Heart /

*"New thoughts and new truths go through three stages.*
*First, they are ridiculed.*
*Next, they are violently opposed.*
*Finally, they are accepted as being self-evident."*

**Arthur Schopenhauer**

Matthias Rath, M.D.

# Why Animals Don't Get Heart Attacks

## ... But People Do!

### The Discovery That Will Eradicate Heart Disease

**The natural prevention of heart attacks, strokes, high blood pressure, diabetes, high cholesterol and many other cardiovascular conditions**

© 2003 MATTHIAS RATH, M.D.
ISBN 0-9679546-8-1

4th Revised Edition

Dr.Rath Education Services USA, BV
1260 Memorex Drive
Suite 100
Santa Clara, CA 95050

1-800-624-2442

www.drrathresearch.org

**This book is not intended as a substitute for the medical advice of a physician.**
The reader should regularly consult a physician in matters relating to his or her health and particularly in respect to any symptoms that may require diagnosis or medical attention. The authors and the publisher disclaim responsibility for any adverse effects resulting directly or indirectly from the information contained in this book.

**RSAP10476**

# Table of Contents

9

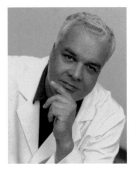

Dear Reader:

The largest "epidemic" on earth is caused by heart attacks, strokes and other forms of cardiovascular disease that have cost hundreds of millions of lives. Today, we know that this "cardiovascular epidemic" is not a genuine disease, but the result of long-term deficiencies of vitamins and other essential nutrients in millions of cells of our bodies — and it is preventable. *This book is an account of this discovery, which will save millions of lives worldwide.*

The "cardiovascular epidemic" is one of the largest economic burdens in America and other countries. The direct and indirect costs associated with this disease amount to trillions of dollars worldwide each year. *This book shows how these funds can be freed for other important public and private tasks.*

This very same "cardiovascular epidemic" is also the core of the largest investment business on earth — the pharmaceutical "business with disease." The end of this epidemic will inevitably terminate the pharmaceutical business as we know it today. *This book is the pharmaceutical industry's "Enemy Number One."*

With the largest and most profitable investment industry on earth fighting the discoveries documented in this book, it is no surprise that you may not have heard about them elsewhere. The drug industry buys influence in the media, medicine and politics, and it has been the largest corporate donor for the current US Administration. *Thus, the faster the message of this book spreads, the sooner the unscrupulous "business with disease" will end.*

The dramatic global changes that eventually followed these discoveries were recognized early on by the two-time Nobel Laureate Linus Pauling. Shortly before his death he told me: "Your discoveries are so important for millions of people that they threaten entire industries. One day there may even be wars just to prevent this breakthrough from being widely accepted. This is the time when you need to stand up!" This is why recently I exposed these corporate interests behind the Iraq War in the *New York Times* and other leading international newspapers.

The global scope of the health benefits from the discoveries documented in this book is breathtaking. Their implementation into national health care policies will significantly reduce and eliminate three leading causes of mortality in the world today: cardiovascular disease, strokes and deaths caused by the side-effects of prescription drugs. *This book provides the guidelines to reach this goal.*

No matter what your age, gender, nationality or income, virtually everyone can benefit immediately from the termination of the pharmaceutical "business with disease." Together, we can save millions of lives and trillions of dollars in health care costs. *This book is a practical guide for what you can do now.*

The "Liberation of Human Health" is the largest liberation movement of all time. Its scope is global and directly affects the health and lives of six billion people inhabiting our planet today, as well as those of future generations. *This book calls upon you to participate in this great mission — in the name of your children and grandchildren.*

The only historical analogy that comes close to this movement is the "liberation from illiteracy" in Medieval Europe. With the invention of the printing press and the translation of the Bible into spoken languages 500 years ago, millions of people took the right to learn to read and write in their own hands. The rulers then knew that "knowledge is power" and they did not want to share it. But millions of people then did not ask for permission. Their common effort terminated the Dark Ages and inaugurated the Modern Times — and the unprecedented progress of mankind.

Today, the "Liberation of Human Health" from the global yoke of the pharmaceutical "business with disease" offers even greater rewards for mankind — among them the eradication of today's most common diseases. But these rewards do not come by themselves. *We all need to work for a world in which health, peace and social justice are the rule — and not the exception. This book will guide you toward this goal.*

Sincerely,

Matthias Rath, MD

11

# Introduction

- The Mission to Eradicate Heart Disease

- How You Can Immediately Benefit From Reading This Book

- Dr. Rath's Ten Step Program for Natural Cardiovascular Health

- Dr. Rath's Cellular Health Recommendations Provide Biological Fuel to Millions of Cells

- Cellular Medicine: The Solution to Cardiovascular Disease

# The Mission to Eradicate Heart Disease

**We, the People of the World, Declare the 21st Century as the "Century of Eradicating Heart Disease."**

**Only once in the course of human events** comes the time when heart attacks, strokes and other cardiovascular conditions are being eradicated. That time is now. Just as the discovery that microorganisms are the cause of infectious diseases led to the control of infectious epidemics, so will the discovery that heart attacks and strokes are the result of long-term vitamin deficiencies lead to the control of the cardiovascular disease epidemic. Mankind can eradicate heart disease as a major cause of death and disability during the 21st century.

**Animals don't get heart attacks** because they produce vitamin C in their bodies, which protects their blood vessel walls. In humans, who are unable to produce vitamin C, dietary vitamin deficiency of this nutrient weakens the blood vessel walls. Cardiovascular disease is an early form of scurvy. Clinical studies document that the optimum daily intake of vitamins and other essential nutrients halts and reverses coronary heart disease naturally. These essential nutrients supply vital bioenergy to millions of heart and blood vessel cells, thereby optimizing cardiovascular function. An optimum supply of vitamins and other essential nutrients can prevent and help correct cardiovascular conditions naturally. Heart attacks, strokes, high blood pressure, irregular heartbeat, heart failure, circulatory problems in diabetes and other cardiovascular problems will be essentially unknown in future generations.

**The eradication of heart disease** is the next great goal uniting all mankind. The availability of vitamins and other essential nutrients needed to control the global cardiovascular disease epidemic is unlimited. The eradication of heart disease is dependent on one single factor: how fast we can spread the message that vitamins and other essential nutrients are the solution to the cardiovascular disease epidemic.

**The main hurdles we have to overcome** are the interests of pharmaceutical companies and other special interest groups, which are trying to block the spread of this lifesaving information in order to protect a global prescription drug market. But the health interests of millions of people are more important than the stock price of any drug company. We, the people of the world, recognize that we have to protect our health interests and that the eradication of heart disease is dependent upon our joint efforts.

**We, the people of all nations,** races and religions; local, regional and national governments; public and private organizations; health insurers, health maintenance organizations, hospitals, medical offices and other health care providers; churches, schools, businesses and other community groups, recognize our historic opportunity and responsibility to act now – for our generation and for all generations to come.

- **We proclaim the 21st century as the "Century of Eradicating Heart Disease."**

- **We will spread information about the lifesaving benefits of vitamins.**

- **We invite everyone to join us in winning one of the greatest victories of mankind.**

> *To my readers: If you read this book and recognize its significance for your own health and for the lives of everyone you know — take action! Share this information with others! Use this "Mission Statement" to show the dimension of global health improvement to others. Start a natural health initiative in your community!*

# One Hundred Years Ago: Eradicating Epidemics

For millennia, infectious diseases were the number one cause of death on earth and billions of people died from them.

For millennia, people believed that the cause of these epidemics was a curse from heaven.

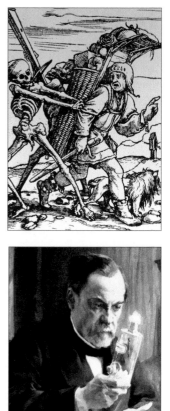

Louis Pasteur discovered that these epidemics were caused by bacteria and other microorganisms.

This discovery enabled the implementation of preventive methods, as well as the development of vaccines and antibiotics.

A few years ago, the World Health Organization (WHO) declared the first infectious disease, smallpox, eradicated.

# Today: Eradicating Heart Disease

During the last century, cardio-vascular disease has become the number one cause of death in the industrialized world. World-wide, over one billion people have died from heart attacks and strokes.

Because the main cause of car-diovascular disease has re-mained unknown until now, the cardiovascular disease epidemic has continued to spread on a global scale.

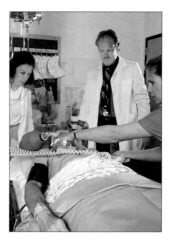

This book documents the scientific discovery that provides the solution to the cardiovascular disease epidemic: Animals don't get heart attacks because – as opposed to humans – they produce vitamin C in their bodies. Thus, heart attacks and strokes are not diseases, but the consequence of chronic vitamin deficiency and, as such, are preventable.

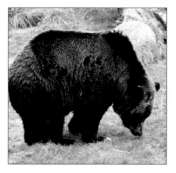

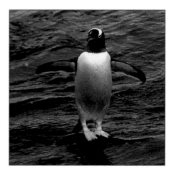

# How You Can Immediately Benefit From Reading This Book

This book summarizes the medical breakthrough in the area of vitamins and cardiovascular health.

**Why animals don't get heart attacks, but every second man and woman dies from them:** Animals don't get heart attacks because they produce large amounts of vitamin C in their bodies. Vitamin C optimizes the production of collagen and other reinforcement molecules, thereby stabilizing the walls of the arteries and preventing atherosclerotic deposits, heart attacks and strokes. We human beings cannot manufacture a single molecule of vitamin C in our bodies and, in addition, almost everyone gets too few vitamins from the diet. The inevitable consequence of this is a weakening of the artery walls, which triggers artery wall deposits (atherosclerosis). Thus, chronic vitamin deficiency — not high cholesterol — is the main cause of the cardiovascular disease epidemic.

**The world's first patented therapy for the natural reversal of cardiovascular disease:** This book presents the world's first patented therapy for the reversal of atherosclerotic deposits without angioplasty or bypass surgery. Once the artery wall is weakened by vitamin deficiency, the body mobilizes its repair mechanisms. Millions of fat particles (lipoproteins) are deposited in the artery wall by means of biological "adhesives," which eventually leads to atherosclerosis, clogging of the arteries, heart attacks and strokes. Atherosclerotic deposits can now be largely prevented and reversed with natural "Teflon" agents, which neutralize these adhesive properties. The first generation of artery wall "Teflon" agents are the natural amino acids lysine and proline, which become even more effective in combination with other vitamins. Thus, an old dream of mankind becomes reality: the natural reversal of cardiovascular disease — without angioplasty or bypass surgery.

**The world's first vitamin program clinically proven to reverse coronary artery disease naturally:** Dr. Rath's Cellular Health recommendations comprise the world's first natural health program to halt and actually reverse existing coronary artery deposits. Drug companies selling cholesterol-lowering drugs and diet prophets have been making similar claims without substantiation. This book documents unequivocally that only a vitamin-based program provides the decisive bioenergy for the cells of the artery walls to initiate the healing process. For the first time in the history of medicine, you will actually see proof that coronary deposits, the cause of heart attacks, can entirely disappear in a natural way. By taking advantage of Dr. Rath's Cellular Health recommendations, physicians and patients alike now have an effective, natural alternative to angioplasty, bypass surgery and other conventional treatments for cardiovascular disease.

**The discoveries documented in this book have led to the world's leading cardiovascular health program:** Dr. Rath's Cellular Health recommendations include a selection of essential vitamins, minerals and natural amino acids used in combination with a healthy lifestyle. These micronutrients provide essential bioenergy for millions of cells composing the cardiovascular system. This essential nutrient program was developed as a daily supplement for men and women of any age to protect the heart and blood vessel system in a natural way. Millions of people worldwide are already following this program for prevention and adjunct therapy. This book documents the profound health benefits of this program in even the most severe health conditions, such as angina pectoris, irregular heartbeat, heart failure, diabetes, high blood pressure, post heart attack and many others. Thus, it is not surprising that Dr. Rath's Cellular Health recommendations have become today's leading cardiovascular health program, and patients around the world are benefiting from it.

**This book is an authentic report of one of the greatest breakthroughs in medicine:** This book is written by the scientist and physician who led this medical advance from its beginning. The last two chapters document the decisive discoveries, the development of an entirely new understanding of the origins of heart disease and the early support of the two-time Nobel Laureate Linus Pauling. You will also read how the scientific discoveries of this book triggered one of the largest battles in the history of the United States — the Battle for Vitamin Freedom." It documents the historic victory millions of Americans gained over the FDA and the pharmaceutical industry. Passage of the Dietary Supplement Health and Education Act (DSHEA) finally allowed health information in connection with vitamins to be freely disseminated.

**This book has unmasked the pharmaceutical industry as an investment industry conducting a trillion dollar "business with disease":** The annual market for cardiovascular prescription drugs in the United States alone surpasses 100 billion dollars. However, these drugs — including beta-blockers, ACE inhibitors, calcium blockers, cholesterol-lowering drugs and many others — merely cover symptoms; they do not target the cellular root cause of the disease. This is neither a surprise nor a coincidence. It is a simple fact that the pharmaceutical industry is an investment industry; its marketplace is the diseases in your body, and the future of this industry depends on the continuation of these diseases. Prevention, root cause cures and, above all, the eradication of diseases threaten the giant financial interests behind this industry.

The discovery that certain micronutrients can prevent and treat cardiovascular diseases at the cellular level poses a fundamental threat to the core of the entire pharmaceutical investment business. Unable to fight the scientific truth of my discoveries and the fact that animals don't get heart attacks because they make their own vitamin C, the pharmaceutical companies have embarked on a worldwide effort to block the spread of this information. Toward this end, the pharmaceutical lobbyists are even abusing the national and international legislative bodies, including the United Nations' "Codex Alimentarius (Food Standards) Commission." Their unethical goal is to outlaw all health statements in relation to natural, non-patentable therapies for all member countries of the United Nations, or worldwide.

**This book is the starting point of a new health care system:** Over the last decade, several million copies of the previous edition of this book have been sold around the world. This book introduces an entirely new understanding of health and disease, which will enable people to take responsibility for their own bodies and health. This book has become the foundation of a new health care system based on the following principles:

- Natural health education for people will replace the unhealthy dependence on pharmaceutical medicine.
- Children will learn in kindergarten and other grades that their bodies do not produce vitamin C and other key nutrients, which they need to supplement for a healthy life.
- Everyone will understand that health and disease are determined, not at the level of organs, but at the level of millions of cells composing the body.
- Every living room will become a consulting center for Cellular Health information.
- The priority for the new health care system is the natural prevention and eradication of diseases.
- Effective, safe and affordable natural therapies will eliminate the trillion dollar, symptom-oriented pharmaceutical "business with disease."
- Patient-oriented and community-based health care will improve health, extend life expectancy and reduce the need for expensive interventional medicine.
- Medical research focused on the prevention and eradication of diseases will replace drug research driven by market shares and shareholder interests.

We invite you to join our Health Alliance to improve your own health, to help your family, friends and colleagues and to start building this new health care system in your own community.

# Dr. Rath's Ten Step Program for Natural Cardiovascular Health

1. **Understand the function of your cardiovascular system.**
   Your blood vessel pipeline system measures 60,000 miles and is the largest organ in your body. Your heart beats 100,000 times every day, performing the greatest amount of work of all organs. Your body is as old as your cardiovascular system, and optimizing your cardiovascular health adds years to your life.

2. **Stabilize the walls of your blood vessels.**
   Blood vessel instability and lesions in your blood vessel walls are the primary causes for cardiovascular disease. Vitamin C is the "cement" of the blood vessel walls and stabilizes them. Animals don't get heart disease because they produce enough endogenous vitamin C in their livers to protect their blood vessels. In contrast, we humans develop deposits in the blood vessel walls that lead to heart attacks and strokes because we cannot manufacture endogenous vitamin C, and generally, get too few vitamins from the diet.

3. **Reverse existing deposits in your arteries without surgery.**
   Cholesterol and fat particles are deposited inside the blood vessel walls by means of biological adhesives. "Teflon"-like agents can prevent this stickiness. The amino acids lysine and proline are nature's Teflon-like agents. Together with vitamin C, they help reverse existing deposits naturally.

4. **Relax your blood vessel walls.**
   Deposits and spasms of the blood vessel walls are the causes of high blood pressure. Dietary supplementation of magnesium (nature's calcium antagonist) and vitamin C relaxes the blood vessel walls and normalizes high blood pressure. The natural amino acid arginine can be of additional benefit.

5. **Optimize the performance of your heart.**
   The heart is the motor of the cardiovascular system. Like the motor of your car, the millions of muscle cells need fuel for

optimum performance. Nature's "cell fuels" include carnitine, coenzyme Q-10, B vitamins and many other nutrients and trace elements. Dietary supplementation of these essential nutrients will optimize the pumping performance of the heart and contribute to a regular heartbeat.

**6. Protect your cardiovascular pipelines from rusting.**
Biological rusting, or oxidation, damages your cardiovascular system and accelerates aging. Vitamin C, vitamin E, beta-carotene and selenium are the most important natural antioxidants. Dietary supplementation of these antioxidants provides important rust protection for your cardiovascular system. Don't smoke because cigarette smoke accelerates the biological rusting of your blood vessels.

**7. Exercise regularly.**
Regular physical activity is a precondition for cardiovascular health. Moderate, regular exercise such as walking or bicycling is ideal, and can be performed by everyone.

**8. Eat a prudent diet.**
The diets of our ancestors thousands of generations ago were rich in plant nutrition and high in fiber and vitamins. These dietary preferences have shaped the metabolism of our bodies today. A diet rich in fruits and vegetables and low in fats and sugars enhances cardiovascular health.

**9. Find time to relax.**
Physical and emotional stressors are cardiovascular risk factors. Schedule time to relax. Be aware that the production of the stress hormone adrenaline uses your body's vitamin C. Long-term physical or emotional stress depletes your body's vitamin pool and requires dietary vitamin supplementation.

**10. Start now.**
The buildup of blood vessel deposits starts as early as the second decade of life. The earlier you start my cardiovascular health program, the more years you will add to your life.

# Dr. Rath's Cellular Health Recommendations

## CELLULAR HEALTH - BASIC RECOMMENDATIONS

Dr. Rath's Basic Cellular Health Recommendations comprise more than 30 vitamins, minerals, amino acids and trace elements. These essential nutrients have been selected based on scientific criteria and their main function as bioenergy providers to the multitude of cells composing the human body. These Basic Cellular Health Recommendations are for everyone — young and old, healthy persons and patients — in order to optimize cardiovascular health and help prevent cardiovascular disease, as well as other health problems. The chart on the adjacent page gives the daily minimum amount of each essential nutrient for a healthy adult person. Patients and people with special nutritional needs may double or triple these amounts.

## CELLULAR HEALTH - SPECIAL RECOMMENDATIONS

For patients with certain advanced health problems, such as coronary heart disease, high blood pressure, diabetes, heart failure and others, *Special Cellular Health Recommendations* were developed in addition to the *Basic Cellular Health Recommendations*. These Special Cellular Health recommendations include certain essential nutrients in higher amounts or in addition to those found in the Basic Cellular Health Recommendations.

The health benefits of this program are documented throughout this book, as well as in the comprehensive testimonial book, *Good Health-Do It Yourself!*

# Basic Cellular Health Recommendations

### VITAMINS

| | | | |
|---|---:|---|---|
| Vitamin C | 600 | - 3,000 | mg |
| Vitamin E (d-alpha-Tocopherol) | 130 | - 600 | IU |
| Beta-carotene | 1,600 | - 8,000 | IU |
| Vitamin B1 (Thiamine) | 5 | - 40 | mg |
| Vitamin B2 (Riboflavin) | 5 | - 40 | mg |
| Vitamin B3 (Nicotinate) | 45 | - 200 | mg |
| Vitamin B5 (Pantothenate) | 40 | - 200 | mg |
| Vitamin B6 (Pyridoxine) | 10 | - 50 | mg |
| Vitamin B12 (Cyanocobalamin) | 20 | - 100 | mcg |
| Vitamin D3 | 100 | - 600 | IU |
| Folic Acid | 90 | - 400 | mcg |
| Biotin | 60 | - 300 | mcg |

### MINERALS

| | | | |
|---|---:|---|---|
| Calcium | 30 | - 150 | mg |
| Magnesium | 40 | - 200 | mg |
| Potassium | 20 | - 90 | mg |
| Phosphate | 10 | - 60 | mg |

### TRACE ELEMENTS

| | | | |
|---|---:|---|---|
| Zinc | 5 | - 30 | mg |
| Manganese | 1 | - 6 | mg |
| Copper | 300 | - 2,000 | mcg |
| Selenium | 20 | - 100 | mcg |
| Chromium | 10 | - 50 | mcg |
| Molybdenum | 4 | - 20 | mcg |

### OTHER IMPORTANT CELLULAR NUTRIENTS

| | | | |
|---|---:|---|---|
| L-Proline | 100 | - 500 | mg |
| L-Lysine | 100 | - 500 | mg |
| L-Carnitine | 30 | - 150 | mg |
| L-Arginine | 40 | - 150 | mg |
| L-Cysteine | 30 | - 150 | mg |
| Inositol | 30 | - 150 | mg |
| Coenzyme Q-10 | 5 | - 30 | mg |
| Pycnogenol | 5 | - 30 | mg |
| Bioflavonoids | 100 | - 450 | mg |

mg = milligrams, mcg = micrograms

# Dr. Rath's Cellular Health Recommendations Provide Biological Fuel to Millions of Cells

Throughout this book, you will read about remarkable health improvements experienced by people following Dr. Rath's Cellular Health recommendations. The scientific basis of these dramatic health improvements is this: the cells in our bodies fulfill a multitude of different functions. Gland cells produce hormones, white blood cells produce antibodies and heart muscle cells generate and conduct biological electricity for the heartbeat. The specific function of each cell is determined by the genetic "software program," the genes located in each cell core.

Despite these different functions, it is important to understand that all cells use the same "cell fuel" — carriers of bioenergy or biocatalysts — for a multitude of biochemical reactions inside these cells. Many of these essential biocatalysts and bioenergy molecules cannot be produced by the body and must be supplemented in our diets on a regular basis. Certain vitamins, amino acids, minerals and trace elements are among the most important essential nutrients for the optimum function of each cell. Without optimum intake of these essential nutrients, the function of millions of cells becomes impaired and diseases develop.

Unfortunately, conventional medicine still does not recognize the decisive role vitamins and other essential nutrients play in optimum cellular function and health. The modern concept of Cellular Medicine fundamentally changes that. In a few years, daily supplementation of scientifically developed Cellular Health recommendations — such as the ones presented in this book — will be a matter of course for everyone, just like eating and drinking.

**Single Cell (Schematic)**

Cellular Production Line
(Endoplasmic Reticulum)

Cellular Core
Central Unit
(Nucleus)

Cellular Power Plant
(Mitochondrium)

# Important Biocatalysts:

- Vitamin C
- Vitamin B1
- Vitamin B2
- Vitamin B3
- Vitamin B5
- Vitamin B6
- Vitamin B12
- Carnitine
- Coenzyme Q-10
- Minerals
- Trace Elements

The metabolic "software program" of each cell is determined exactly by the genetic information located in each cell core.

Essential nutrients are needed as biocatalysts and carriers of bioenergy in each cell. These functions are essential for the optimum performance of millions of cells.

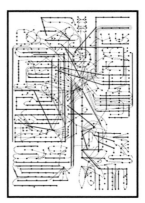

*Dr. Rath's Cellular Health recommendations provide biological fuel to millions of cells.*

27

# Cellular Medicine: The Solution to Cardiovascular Disease

The most profound impact of Cellular Medicine will be in the area of cardiovascular health because the cardiovascular system is the most active organ system of our bodies and, therefore, has the highest consumption of essential nutrients. The image on the opposite page illustrates the most important cells of the cardiovascular system.

**The cells of the blood vessel walls:** The endothelial cells form the barrier or protective layer between the blood and the blood vessel wall; moreover, these cells contribute to a variety of metabolic functions, such as optimum blood viscosity. The smooth muscle cells produce collagen and other reinforcement molecules, providing optimum stability and tone to the blood vessel walls.

**The blood cells:** Even the millions of blood corpuscles circulating in the bloodstream are nothing other than cells. They are responsible for oxygen transport, defense, scavenging, wound healing and many other functions. The following pages describe how deficiencies in vitamins and other essential nutrients in these different cell types are closely associated with the most frequent cardiovascular diseases today.

**The cells of the heart muscle:** The main role of heart muscle cells is the pumping function to maintain blood circulation. A subtype of heart muscle cell is specialized and capable of generating and conducting biological electricity for the heartbeat.

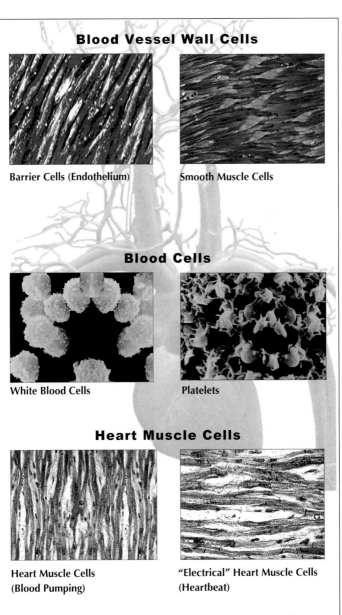

# Blood Vessel Wall Cells

Barrier Cells (Endothelium)

Smooth Muscle Cells

# Blood Cells

White Blood Cells

Platelets

# Heart Muscle Cells

Heart Muscle Cells
(Blood Pumping)

"Electrical" Heart Muscle Cells
(Heartbeat)

*The cardiovascular system is composed of millions of cells.*

29

# Vitamin Deficiency in Artery Wall Cells Causes Heart Attacks, Strokes and High Blood Pressure

Long-term deficiency of vitamins and other essential nutrients in millions of vascular wall cells impairs the function of the blood vessel walls. The most frequent consequences of this are high blood pressure conditions and the development of athero-sclerotic deposits, which lead to heart attacks and strokes.

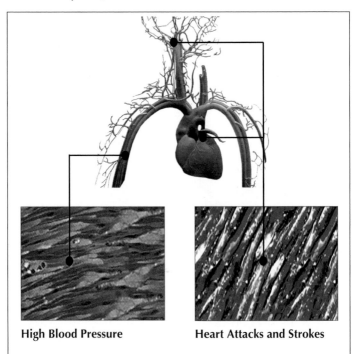

**High Blood Pressure**

Vitamin deficiencies in artery wall cells can lead to:

- Increased artery wall tension
- Narrowing of artery diameter
- Thickening of artery walls and high blood pressure

**Heart Attacks and Strokes**

Vitamin deficiencies in artery wall cells can lead to:

- Instability of artery wall
- Lesion and cracks
- Atherosclerotic deposits, heart attacks and strokes

# Vitamin Deficiency in Heart Muscle Cells Causes Irregular Heartbeat and Heart Failure

A chronic deficiency of vitamins and other essential nutrients in millions of heart muscle cells can contribute to impaired heart function. The most frequent consequences of this are irregular heartbeat (arrhythmia) and heart failure (shortness of breath, edema and fatigue).

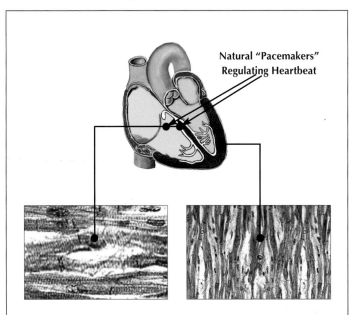

Natural "Pacemakers" Regulating Heartbeat

**Irregular Heartbeat**

Vitamin deficiencies in "electrical" heart muscle cells can lead to:

• Impaired creation and conduction of electrical impulse for heartbeat

• Irregular heartbeat (arrhythmia)

**Heart Failure**

Vitamin deficiencies in heart muscle cells can lead to:

• Impaired blood pumping

• Shortness of breath, edema and severe fatigue

# Notes

# 2

# Atherosclerosis, Heart Attack and Stroke

## Dr. Rath's Cellular Health Recommendations for Prevention and Adjunct Therapy

- The Facts About Coronary Heart Disease

- Dr. Rath's Cellular Health Recommendations:
  - Documented Health Benefits in Patients
  - Documented Health Benefits in Clinical Studies

- Scientific Background Information

# The Facts About Coronary Heart Disease

- **Every second man and woman** in the industrialized world dies from the consequences of atherosclerotic deposits in the coronary arteries (leading to heart attack) or in the arteries supplying blood to the brain (leading to stroke). The epidemic spread of these cardiovascular diseases is largely due to the fact that, until now, the true nature of atherosclerosis and coronary heart disease has been insufficiently understood.

- **Conventional medicine** is largely confined to treating the symptoms of this disease. Calcium antagonists, beta-blockers, nitrates and other drugs are prescribed to alleviate angina pain. Surgical procedures (angioplasty and bypass surgery) are applied to improve blood flow mechanically. Rarely does conventional medicine target the underlying problem: the instability of the vascular wall, which triggers the development of atherosclerotic deposits.

- **Cellular Medicine** provides a breakthrough in our understanding of the underlying causes of these conditions and leads to the effective prevention and treatment of coronary heart disease. The primary cause of coronary heart disease and other forms of atherosclerotic disease is a chronic deficiency of vitamins and other essential nutrients in millions of vascular wall cells. This leads to the instability of the vascular walls, lesions and cracks, atherosclerotic deposits and, eventually, heart attacks or strokes. Since the primary cause of cardiovascular disease is a deficiency of essential nutrients in the vascular wall, the daily optimum intake of these essential nutrients is the primary measure to prevent atherosclerosis and help repair artery wall damage.

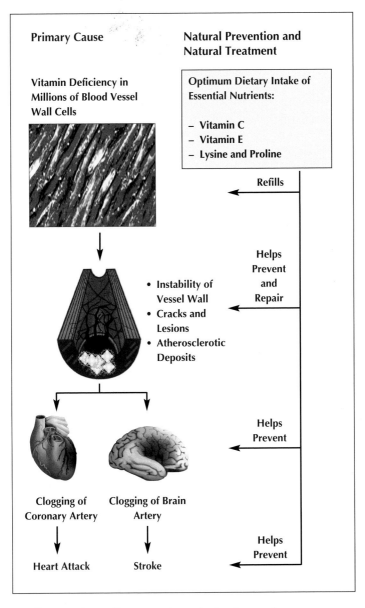

**Primary Cause**

**Natural Prevention and Natural Treatment**

**Vitamin Deficiency in Millions of Blood Vessel Wall Cells**

**Optimum Dietary Intake of Essential Nutrients:**

– **Vitamin C**
– **Vitamin E**
– **Lysine and Proline**

**Refills**

- Instability of Vessel Wall
- Cracks and Lesions
- Atherosclerotic Deposits

**Helps Prevent and Repair**

**Clogging of Coronary Artery**

**Clogging of Brain Artery**

**Helps Prevent**

**Heart Attack**

**Stroke**

**Helps Prevent**

*Coronary heart disease, stroke and other forms of atherosclerotic cardiovascular disease*

35

- **Scientific research and clinical studies** have already documented the particular value of vitamin C, vitamin E, beta-carotene, lysine, proline and other ingredients in Dr. Rath's Cellular Health recommendations for preventing cardiovascular disease and improving the health of patients with existing cardiovascular disease.

- **Dr. Rath's Cellular Health recommendations** comprise specific essential nutrients that help prevent cardiovascular disease naturally and repair existing damage. The following pages document health improvements in patients with coronary heart disease and other forms of cardiovascular disease who have benefited from this program.

- **My recommendation for patients** with cardiovascular disease: Start immediately with this natural cardiovascular program and inform your doctor about it. Follow the Cellular Health recommendations and take your medication. Vitamins C and E are natural "blood thinners." If you are on blood thinning medication, you should talk to your doctor about the vitamins you take so that additional blood tests can be performed and your prescription medication decreased. Do not adjust any medication without consulting your doctor.

- **Prevention is better than treatment.** The success of these Cellular Health recommendations in patients with existing atherosclerosis and cardiovascular disease is based on the fact that the millions of cardiovascular cells are replenished with "cell fuel" for optimum cell function. A natural cardiovascular program proven to correct an existing health condition is, of course, your best choice in preventing this condition in the first place.

# Dr. Rath's Cellular Health Recommendations Can Halt and Reverse Coronary Heart Disease

Millions of people die every year from heart attacks because no effective treatment to halt or reverse coronary heart disease has been available. Therefore, we decided to test the efficacy of Dr. Rath's Cellular Health recommendations for the number one health problem of our time: coronary atherosclerosis, the cause of heart attacks. If these Cellular Health recommendations were able to stop further progression of coronary atherosclerosis, the fight against heart attacks could be won and the goal of eradicating heart disease would become a reality.

To measure the success of this program, we did not primarily look at risk factors circulating in the bloodstream. We focused directly on the key problem, the atherosclerotic deposits inside the walls of the coronary arteries. A fascinating new diagnostic technique had just become available that allowed us to measure the size of the coronary deposits non-invasively: Ultrafast Computed Tomography (Ultrafast CT).

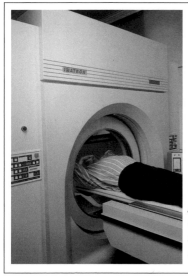

*Ultrafast CT, the "mammogram for the heart," is a new diagnostic technology that allows non-invasive testing for coronary heart disease.*

37

Ultrafast CT measures the area and density of calcium deposits without the use of needles or radioactive dye. The computer automatically calculates their size by determining the Coronary Artery Scan (CAS) score. The higher the CAS score, the more calcium has accumulated, which indicates more advanced coronary heart disease.

Compared to angiography and treadmill tests, Ultrafast CT is the most precise diagnostic technique available today to detect coronary heart disease already in its early stages. This diagnostic test allows the detection of deposits in the coronary arteries long before a patient notices angina pectoris or other symptoms. Moreover, since it directly measures the deposits in the artery walls, Ultrafast CT is a much better indicator of a per-

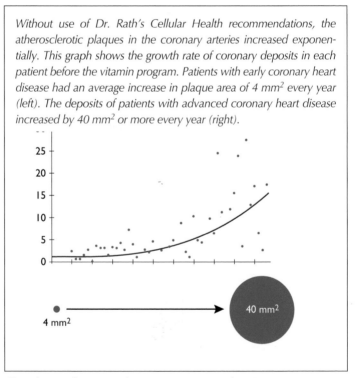

*Without use of Dr. Rath's Cellular Health recommendations, the atherosclerotic plaques in the coronary arteries increased exponentially. This graph shows the growth rate of coronary deposits in each patient before the vitamin program. Patients with early coronary heart disease had an average increase in plaque area of 4 mm² every year (left). The deposits of patients with advanced coronary heart disease increased by 40 mm² or more every year (right).*

*Growth rate of coronary deposits per year in each patient*

son's cardiovascular risk than measurements of cholesterol or other risk factors in the bloodstream.

We studied 55 patients with various degrees of coronary heart disease. Changes in the size of the coronary artery calcifications in each patient were measured over an average period of one year without vitamin supplementation, followed by one year with Dr. Rath's Cellular Health recommendations. In this way, the heart scans of the same person could be compared before and after the vitamin program. This study design had the advantage of patients serving as their own controls. The dosages of essential nutrients given were in the approximate amounts listed in the vitamin table on page 25.

*With use of Dr. Rath's Cellular Health recommendations, the fast growth of coronary artery deposits was slowed during the first six months and essentially stopped during the second six months. As a result, no heart attack would occur. These are the study results of patients with early coronary deposits who, like millions of adults in the prime of their lives, have developed heart disease without yet experiencing symptoms.*

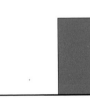

**Monthly growth of coronary deposits <u>before</u> Cellular Health recommendations**

**Monthly growth of coronary deposits: Months 0 - 6 with Cellular Health recommendations**

**Monthly growth of coronary deposits: Months 7 - 12 with Cellular Health recommendations**

*Dr. Rath's Cellular Health recommendations can stop coronary heart disease.*

The results of this study were published in the *Journal of Applied Nutrition*. The full text of this landmark study is documented at the end of this book. The most important findings can be summarized as follows: This study measured, for the first time, how aggressive coronary heart disease progresses until eventually a heart attack occurs. Without the use of Cellular Health recommendations, the coronary calcifications increased at an exponential rate (very fast) with an average growth of 44% every year. Thus, without vitamin protection,

---

*These pictures document a milestone in medicine — the complete natural disappearance of coronary heart disease. The Ultrafast Computed Tomography (Ultrafast CT) scans (top row) document atherosclerotic deposits in the right and left coronary arteries of this patient. After one year with Dr. Rath's Cellular Health recommendations, these coronary deposits entirely disappeared (bottom row)— indicating a natural healing process of the artery wall.*

**Without Vitamin Program**

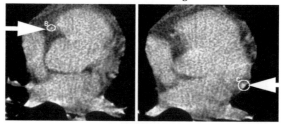

**Deposits in left and right coronary arteries**

**With Vitamin Program**

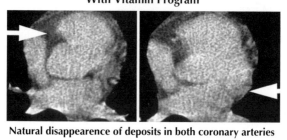

**Natural disappearence of deposits in both coronary arteries**

---

*Dr. Rath's Cellular Health recommendations — the world's first natural therapy documenting the disappearance of coronary deposits*

40

coronary deposits increased approximately half their size every year. When patients followed the Cellular Health recommendations, this trend was reversed and the average growth rate of coronary calcifications actually slowed down. Most significantly, in patients with early stages of the disease, this essential nutrient program stopped further progression of coronary heart disease within one year. This study also gives us valuable information about the time it takes for the Cellular Health recommendations to show a repair effect on the artery wall. While for the first six months the deposits in these patients continued to grow, albeit at a decreased pace, the growth essentially stopped during the second six months with the vitamin program. Of course, any therapy that stops coronary heart disease in its early stages prevents heart attacks later on.

It is not surprising that there is a delay of several months until the healing effect of these Cellular Health recommendations

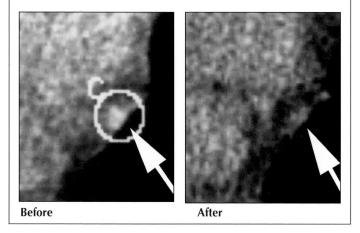

*Before following Dr. Rath's Cellular Health recommendations, the patient had developed atherosclerotic deposits in the walls of his left coronary artery (white circled area in the left picture). The scans below are magnifications of the heart scan taken with Ultrafast CT.*

**Before**                    **After**

*Natural healing of coronary artery disease (magnified)*

41

on the artery wall becomes noticeable. Atherosclerotic deposits develop over many years or decades, and it takes several months to control this aggressive disease and start the healing process. More advanced stages of coronary heart disease may take still longer before the vascular healing process is measurable. To determine this, we are continuing our study.

Can already existing coronary deposits be reversed in a natural way? The answer is yes. In individual patients, we documented the natural reversal and complete disappearance of early coronary artery deposits approximately within one year. The ongoing study will tell us how long the natural reversal takes in patients with advanced coronary artery disease.

The complete natural disappearance of atherosclerotic deposits with Dr. Rath's Cellular Health recommendations confirms that this vitamin program contains the essential ingredients needed to start the natural healing process of the artery wall.

In patients with *early* coronary heart disease, this healing of the artery wall can lead to the complete, natural disapearance of atherosclerotic deposits (see pages 40-41).

In patients with *advanced* coronary artery disease, these Cellular Health recommendations can stabilize the artery walls, halt the further growth of coronary deposits, reverse them, at least in part, and contribute to the prevention of heart attacks.

# Improving Human Health Worldwide

Our clinical study marks a major breakthrough in medicine and will lead to health improvements for millions of people throughout the world. For the first time, the following clinical results were documented:

- Without vitamin therapy, coronary heart disease is a very aggressive disease. Deposits grow, on average, at a staggering rate of 44% per year.

- Dr. Rath's Cellular Health recommendations are proven to halt coronary atherosclerosis, the cause of heart attacks, already in its early stages.

- There now exists an effective natural therapy to prevent and reverse coronary heart disease naturally – without angioplasty, bypass surgery or cholesterol-lowering drugs.

- Every man and woman in any country of the world can immediately take advantage of this medical breakthrough.

- In the coming decades, deaths from heart attacks and strokes will be reduced to a fraction of their current rates, and cardiovascular disease will essentially be unknown to future generations.

# How Dr. Rath's Cellular Health Recommendations Can Help Patients With Coronary Heart Disease

These pages present letters from coronary heart disease patients who have followed my Cellular Health recommendations. This essential nutrient program improved the health of these patients and their quality of life beyond anything possible before.

*Dear Dr. Rath:*

*In August 1990, at the age of 20, I was diagnosed with viral cardiomyopathy. My doctors informed me that my only hope for survival would be a heart transplant. In November 1990, I was transported to the hospital for **heart transplant surgery.***

*As part of my post-operative treatment, I went into the hospital for an annual heart catheterization. Up until January, my heart caths were fine. In January, I had a heart catheterization and my cardiologist found four blockages. **Three (coronary artery) vessels were approximately 90% occluded (blocked) and the fourth vessel was approximately 60% occluded.** I had also gained 100 pounds since the transplant, and my cardiologist was furious. I was instructed to begin a strict, low-fat diet immediately.*

*In May, I was introduced to your Cellular Health recommendations. I had lost 30 pounds on my low-fat diet and began using your formulas. **I had a repeat catheterization in November. The results were phenomenal!! This cath showed that the three occlusions previously at approximately 90% were reduced by approximately 50% and the fourth occlusion previously at approximately 60% had no obstruction at all.** The other exciting news was that I had also lost an additional 50 pounds for a total of 80 pounds!! All of this occurred in six months. This program has dramatically improved my life!*

*Sincerely,*
*J.B.*

*Dear Dr. Rath:*

*I'm a 51-year-old business executive. Because of my position, I am consistently placed in high stress situations. My lifestyle and business responsibilities have caused me to be concerned about the potential of developing coronary artery disease.*

*Approximately two years ago, I scheduled myself for a coronary artery scan on an Ultrafast CT scanner. This new diagnostic technique allows the measurement of small calcifications in the coronary arteries that are invariably associated with atherosclerotic plaques. The test was fast, painless, and involved no injections or any discomfort.*

*My coronary artery scan of two years ago and a second scan one year later showed the **beginnings of atherosclerosis in my coronary arteries.** A few months after my second scan was taken, I was introduced to your vitamin-based cardiovascular health program. After eight months of following your program, I received an additional coronary artery scan in order to evaluate the possible effect of your program on the calcium deposits in my coronary arteries. This most recent coronary artery scan showed that the **calcifications in my coronary arteries had disappeared entirely. It was apparent to me that these deposits had been reversed, or eliminated, during your cardiovascular health program**.*

*Because I was skeptical of the dramatic results, I scheduled a second follow-up coronary artery scan immediately after receiving the results. This follow-up scan confirmed the earlier results, demonstrating no evidence of coronary artery calcification. I must also add that I have made no other significant changes in other aspects of my lifestyle during the past eight months - only your cardiovascular vitamin program. I want to offer you my sincere thanks.*

*Yours truly,*
*S.L.M.*

*Dear Dr. Rath:*

*I am a 57-year-old man, and have lived a very active life. Two years ago, I was diagnosed with* **angina pectoris.** *The cardiologist prescribed a calcium antagonist and nitroglycerin tablets, as needed, for pain. Dr. Rath, I was taking 8-10 nitroglycerin tablets weekly.*

*Then I was introduced to your Cellular Health recommendations and a fiber formula, and within 6 weeks I no longer needed the nitroglycerin. I was not able to mow my yard with a push mower without stopping every 5 to 10 minutes to take a nitroglycerin tablet.* **About a week ago, I push-mowed my entire yard, about three hours of work. I did not stop at all and did not have any chest pain. I felt great.** *I have also lost about 10 pounds, and my cholesterol level dropped from 274 to 191. My doctor says he is real pleased with my condition.*

*I am indebted to you for a great change in my life. With your help, I will be able to live a more fulfilling life for a longer time for a lot less money.*

*Thank you so very much.*
*H.D.*

---

*Dear Dr. Rath:*

*I am an 85-year-old woman. Ten years ago, I was diagnosed with angina pectoris.* **I was told by my doctor that two major arteries were 95% blocked.** *The doctor prescribed nitroglycerin tablets to relieve the painful condition induced by stress. I have been taking three nitroglycerin tablets a day for chest pains for 10 years.*

**Last December, I started on your cardiovascular vitamin program. After two months, I was almost completely off nitroglycerin,** *and now I take a nitroglycerin tablet only occasionally.*

*Sincerely,*
*R.A.*

*Dear Dr. Rath:*

*In July, I complained of chest pain and pain in my left arm. During a treadmill test of about 9 minutes, I had pain in my chest and numbness in my left arm. I was given nitroglycerin, and the pain went away immediately. The following day I was admitted to the hospital for an angiogram. The doctor also found that I had an overactive thyroid.*

***The results of the angiogram indicated that my left main (coronary) artery was 75% blocked and that I would need a double bypass.*** *The doctors didn't want to do the surgery until my thyroid condition was under control.*

*In the meantime, I started your Cellular Health recommendations. I tripled the dosage, while continuing to take the doctor's prescribed medication. The heart surgeon called me for open heart surgery even though my thyroid condition was not yet under control.* ***When the cardiologist set up a thallium treadmill test, he was amazed by the results – they were normal, with no chest pain or shortness of breath. He told me that I could postpone the surgery indefinitely and come back in six months.***

*Just last week the doctor looked at my laboratory records and said, "This is amazing." He went across the hall to see the cardiologist to make sure the report was correct.*

*Thank you again, Dr. Rath. I think this is the beginning of the end of heart disease.*

*Sincerely,*
*J.K.*

*Dear Dr. Rath:*

*I was very excited about the possibility of improving heart function and reversing heart disease due to atherosclerosis after reading your books this past February. **I have familial hypercholesterolemia (high cholesterol), and had a myocardial infarction six years ago at age 40.***

*I started following your cardiovascular vitamin program and using a fiber formula in February. Within the first month, I started feeling less tired, and was able to keep on going without exhaustion or angina. Within two months, the pain in my lower left leg, due to poor circulation (atherosclerosis), disappeared. My heart feels like it's just on overdrive - just purring along - no longer pounding in my chest.*

*My annual physical in May was quite interesting. I never told my doctor I was doing anything different, but he shared with me that my ECG looked normal! **I asked my doctor about possibly lowering my heart medication (a calcium antagonist and beta-blocker). He said that based on my examination he would take me off all this medicine** if I lost 17 more pounds of weight. I have already lost 12 pounds since February, so I see losing 17 pounds as just a matter of time.*

*I have supplemented your vitamin program with additional vitamin C, L-proline, and L-lysine. I do not know if my atherosclerosis will ever be 100% reversed, but I do know that whatever progress your program has brought me so far has already improved my condition, and has impacted my overall quality of life.*

*I will continue your cardiovascular health program for the rest of my life, and I recommend it to anyone concerned about their health.*

*I thank God for your research.*

*Sincerest regards,*
*R.R.*

*Dear Dr. Rath:*

*I am a 57-year-old male who had a heart attack on November 20, 1986.* **I was told by my cardiologist that I had incurred a myocardial infarction** *of a small artery in the lower portion of my heart. It was determined that angioplasty or some other surgical procedure was not relevant or pertinent. The aftereffects were reduced energy and stamina, angina pectoris and other related symptoms typical of this condition. Since that time, I have been on a calcium antagonist medication. Follow-up angioplasty procedures were performed in October 1987 and February 1993. Evidence of a noticeable change in my condition was limited to some increase in the partial blockage in other major coronary arteries.*

*I began following your Cellular Health recommendations last October. This April, another angioplasty was performed on me by a cardiologist who is highly respected and has many years of experience in this specialty area. He has performed several thousand of these procedures; however, he was amazed at what he observed in my case.* **He found the previously blocked artery to have 25% to 30% blood flow and no advancement in the partial obstruction (blocking) of other arteries.** *His comment was, "Your arteries look great. I don't know what you are doing, but keep doing it."* **He further commented that this was only the second time he had observed an artery opening up that was previously blocked without some surgical procedure.**

*I have experienced a remarkable improvement in my general health by a reduction in the incidence of angina, chest pressure, shortness of breath, and, I have increased energy and endurance. I truly believe your cardiovascular health program will extend my life and eliminate what appeared to be the inevitable need for cardiac bypass surgery some time in the future. Your program has dramatically improved my life, and I am very grateful.*

*Sincerely,*
*L.T.*

*Dear Dr. Rath:*

*A friend of mine started on your Cellular Health recommendations because of minor heart problems. I did not know, but he was also* **scheduled for eye surgery because of a blood vessel blockage.** *He went into the hospital for surgery last week. The doctor looked into his eyes and couldn't believe what he saw.*

**His blockages had cleared, and he no longer needed the surgery done!** *Needless to say, he has been telling everyone he knows about your cardiovascular health program.*

*Sincerely,*
*C.Z.*

A growing number of health professionals around the world are suggesting my Cellular Health recommendations to their patients as an adjunct therapy. They appreciate that, finally, a clinically tested, natural health program is available. The benefits are evident from the following letter from a patient to his doctor:

*Dear Doctor:*

*I can't wait to see you in six weeks. Since following Dr. Rath's Cellular Health recommendations, I have had no angina. This past month, I have walked and climbed the rugged trails of the rain forest without so much as a twinge. And recently, I have walked the last two to 18 holes of a golf course, something unheard of since my heart attack. In closing, my family and I are very pleased, and would like to thank you.*

*Sincerely,*
*J.T.*

# Clinical Studies Document the Prevention of Cardiovascular Disease With Vitamins

The paramount importance of several components of my Cellular Health recommendations in the prevention of cardiovascular disease has also been documented in numerous clinical and epidemiological studies.

Dr. James Enstrom and his colleagues at the University of California at Los Angeles investigated the vitamin intake of more than 11,000 Americans over a period of 10 years. This government-supported study showed that people who consumed at least 300 mg per day of vitamin C through their diet or in the form of nutritional supplements, compared to 50 mg contained in the average American diet, could reduce their heart disease risk up to 50% in men and up to 40% in women. The same study showed that a higher intake of vitamin C was associated with an increased life expectancy of up to six years.

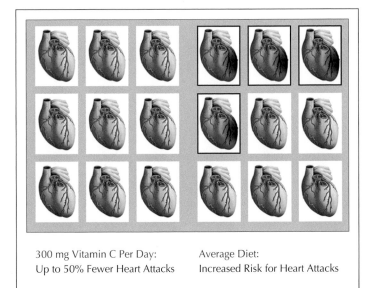

300 mg Vitamin C Per Day:
Up to 50% Fewer Heart Attacks

Average Diet:
Increased Risk for Heart Attacks

*Vitamin C cuts risk for heart attacks in half.*

51

The Canadian physician Dr. G.C. Willis showed that dietary vitamin C can reverse atherosclerosis. At the beginning of his study, he documented the atherosclerotic deposits in his patients by angiography (injection of a radioactive substance followed by X-ray pictures). After this documentation, half of the study patients received 1.5 grams of vitamin C per day. The other half of the patients received no additional vitamin C. The control analysis, on average, after 10-12 months showed in patients who had received additional vitamin C that the atherosclerotic deposits had decreased in 30% of the cases. In contrast, no decrease in atherosclerotic deposits could be seen in those patients who had not received vitamin C supplementation. The deposits in these patients either had remained the same or had increased further.

Amazingly, this important clinical study was not followed up for half a century, and 12 million people continued to die each year from this preventable disease!

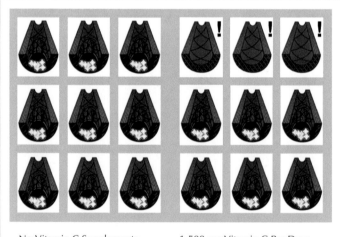

No Vitamin C Supplements:
Coronary Deposits Grow

1,500 mg Vitamin C Per Day:
Halt and Reversal of Deposits
in 30% of Patients

# Europe: More Vitamins — Less Heart Disease

One of the largest studies about the importance of vitamins in the prevention of cardiovascular disease was conducted in Europe. It is a well-known fact that cardiovascular diseases are more frequent in Scandinavia and northern European countries, compared to Mediterranean countries.

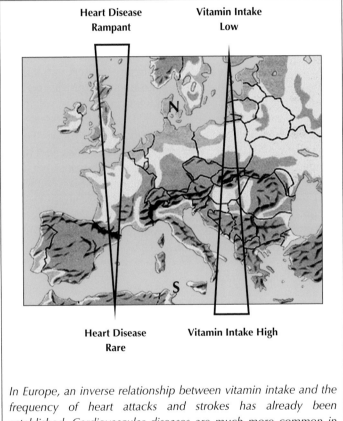

*In Europe, an inverse relationship between vitamin intake and the frequency of heart attacks and strokes has already been established. Cardiovascular diseases are much more common in northern European countries where vitamin intake is low. However, people in Mediterranean countries enjoy a diet rich in vitamins and, consequently, cardiovascular diseases are rare.*

Professor K.F. Gey, from the University of Berne in Switzerland, compared the rate of cardiovascular disease in these countries to the blood levels of vitamin C and beta-carotene, as well as cholesterol. His findings were remarkable:

- People in northern European countries have the highest rate of cardiovascular disease and, on average, the lowest blood levels of vitamins.

- Southern European populations have the lowest cardiovascular risk and the highest blood levels of vitamins.

- An optimum intake of the vitamins C, E and A had a much greater impact on decreasing the risk for cardiovascular disease than lowering cholesterol levels.

This study finally provides the scientific answer to the "French Phenomenon" and the low rate of heart attacks in France, Greece and other Mediterranean countries. The decisive factor for the low cardiovascular risk in these countries is an optimum intake of vitamins in the regular diets of these regions. Certain dietary preferences, such as the consumption of wine and olive oil, which are rich in bioflavonoids and vitamin E seem to be of particular importance.

# Cellular Health Recommendations Clinically Proven to Decrease Your Cardiovascular Disease Risk

Optimum dietary intake of vitamin E, beta-carotene and certain other essential nutrients also significantly reduce cardiovascular disease risk. In clinical and epidemiological (population) studies, the importance of these vitamins for optimum cardiovascular health has been documented:

**The Nurses' Health Study included more than 87,000 American nurses, ages 34-59:** None of the study participants had any signs of cardiovascular disease at the beginning of the study. In 1993, a first result was published in the *New England Journal of Medicine*. It was shown that study participants taking more than 200 International Units of vitamin E per day could reduce their risk for heart attacks by 34%, compared to those receiving only three International Units, which corresponded to the average daily intake of vitamin E in America.

**The Health Professional Study included more than 39,000 health professionals, ages 40-75:** At the beginning of the study, none of the participants had any signs of cardiovascular disease, diabetes or elevated blood cholesterol levels. The study showed that people taking 400 International Units of vitamin E per day could reduce their risk for heart attack by 40%, compared to those taking only six International Units of vitamin E per day. In the same study, an increased intake of beta-carotene was also shown to significantly decrease cardiovascular disease risk.

**The Physicians' Health Study included more than 22,000 physicians, ages 40-84:** In this study in patients with existing cardiovascular disease published by Dr. Charles Hennekens in 1992, it was shown that in those patients, 50 mg of beta-carotene per day could cut the risk for suffering a heart attack or stroke in half.

**The Cambridge Heart Antioxidant Study with vitamin E:** In this study, participants with existing atherosclerosis who received either 400 or 800 International Units of vitamin E suffered 47% fewer non-fatal heart attacks than participants who received a placebo. In their review of several clinical studies, authors David H. Emmert, MD and Jeffrey T. Kirchner, DO noted that cardiovascular mortality could be reduced with the use of vitamin E.

**A multi-center study showed decreased risk for coronary heart disease, stroke and peripheral vascular disease with higher levels of folic acid, and vitamin B6 and vitamin B12:** In a clinical study with more than 1,500 patients, Dr. K. Robinson from the Cleveland Clinic Foundation in Ohio showed that blood levels of vitamin B6, vitamin B12 and folic acid are important in lowering homocysteine levels and decreasing the risk of coronary heart disease.

**A large-scale study in Finland showed that optimum vitamin C intake is the single most important factor for preventing strokes in high blood pressure patients:** In a 10-year study with more than 2,400 patients who were overweight and suffered from high blood pressure, it was shown that low levels of vitamin C increased the risk for a stroke by almost threefold. This study was conducted by Dr. Sudhir Kurl and his colleagues at the University of Kuopio in Finland.

**A 20-year study in Japan showed that optimum vitamin C intake is the single most important factor for preventing all forms of strokes in men and women:** In a clinical study involving more than 2,000 patients over two decades, Dr. Tetsuji Yokoyama and his colleagues from the University of Tokyo, Japan found that high vitamin C levels are the most important factor in determining whether men and women aged 40 and older would suffer a stroke later in life.

---

No prescription drug has ever been shown to be as effective as the components of Dr. Rath's Cellular Health recommendations in preventing coronary heart disease and strokes.

---

# Cellular Health Recommendations for Patients With Coronary Heart Disease

**In addition to my Basic Cellular Health Recommendations (page 25), I recommend that patients with existing coronary heart disease or a high risk for this condition take the following cellular micronutrients in higher dosages.**

- **Vitamin C:** provides protection and the natural healing of the artery wall and reversal of plaques

- **Vitamin E:** provides antioxidant protection

- **Vitamin D:** optimizes calcium metabolism and the reversal of calcium deposits in the artery wall

- **Folic acid:** provides a protective function against increased homocysteine levels together with vitamin B6, vitamin B12 and biotin

- **Biotin:** provides a protective function against increased homocysteine levels together with vitamin B6, vitamin B12 and folic acid

- **Copper:** supports stability of the artery wall with the improved cross-linking of collagen molecules

- **Proline:** supports collagen production, stability of the artery wall and reversal of plaques

- **Lysine:** supports collagen production, stability of the artery wall and reversal of plaques

- **Chondroitin sulfate:** supports the stability of the artery wall as a "cement" for connective tissue

- **N-acetyl-glucosamine:** supports the stability of the artery wall as a "cement" for connective tissue

- **Pycnogenol:** acts as a biocatalyst for improved vitamin C function and improved stability of the artery wall

# Scientific Background for Dr. Rath's Cellular Health Recommendations in Cardiovascular Disease

## What Is Atherosclerosis?

The images on this page are cross-sections of the coronary arteries of a patient with coronary artery disease. These images provide a look inside these arteries through a microscope. The dark ring you notice is the original blood vessel wall as it would be found in a newborn baby. The gray area within this dark ring indicates atherosclerotic deposits, which developed over many years.

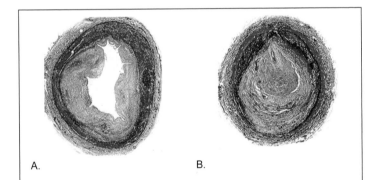

A.                                          B.

*Picture A shows atherosclerotic deposits in coronary arteries, which reduce blood flow and impair oxygen and nutrient supply to millions of heart muscle cells. The coronary arteries of patients with angina pectoris typically look like this.*

*Picture B shows the coronary arteries of a patient who died from a heart attack. On top of the atherosclerotic deposits, a blood clot formed and completely interrupted the blood flow through this artery. This is called a heart attack. Millions of heart muscle cells die, leaving the heart muscle permanently impaired or causing the death of the patient.*

It is important to understand that the atherosclerotic deposits in Picture A developed over many years. In contrast, the additional blood clot in Picture B developed within minutes or perhaps seconds. The effective prevention of heart attacks has to start as early as possible with the prevention of atherosclerotic deposits. Atherosclerosis is not a disease of just those advanced in age. Studies of soldiers killed in the Korean and Vietnam Wars showed that nearly 75% of the victims had already developed some form of atherosclerotic deposits by age 25 or younger. The picture below shows the coronary artery of a 25-year-old victim of a traffic accident. This coincidental finding shows how far atherosclerosis can advance in young adults – without causing any symptoms.

The main cause of atherosclerotic deposits is the biological weakness of the artery walls caused by chronic vitamin deficiency. The atherosclerotic deposits are the consequence of this chronic weakness; they develop as a compensatory stabilizing cast of nature to strengthen weakened blood vessel walls.

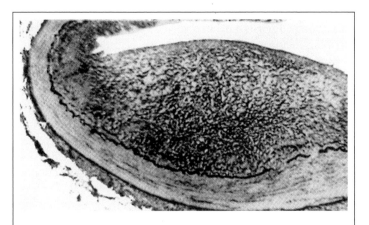

*A cross-section (magnified) of the coronary artery of a 25-year-old victim of a traffic accident. The atherosclerotic deposits had developed without the young man's knowledge.*

# Why Animals Don't Get Heart Attacks

According to the statistics of the World Health Organization, each year more than 12 million people die from the consequences of heart attacks and strokes. Amazingly, while cardiovascular disease has become one of the largest epidemics ever to haunt mankind, these very same heart attacks are essentially unknown in the animal world. The following paragraph from the renowned textbook of veterinary medicine, V*eterinary Pathology* by T.C. Jones and H.A. Smith, documents these facts:

> *"The fact remains, however, that in none of the domestic species, with the rarest of exceptions, do animals develop atherosclerotic disease of clinical significance. It appears that most of the pertinent pathological mechanisms operate in animals and that atherosclerotic disease in them is not impossible;* **it just does not occur.** *If the reason for this could be found, it might cast some very useful light on the human disease."*

These important observations were first published in 1958. Now, more than four decades later, the puzzle of human cardiovascular disease has been solved. The solution to the puzzle of human cardiovascular disease is one of the greatest advances in medicine.

Here is the main reason why animals don't get heart attacks: With few exceptions, animals produce vitamin C in their bodies. The daily amounts of vitamin C produced by animals vary between 1,000 mg and 20,000 mg, compared to human body weight. Vitamin C is the "cement" of the artery wall, and optimum amounts of vitamin C stabilize the arteries. In contrast, we human beings cannot produce a single molecule of vitamin C ourselves. Our ancestors lost this ability generations ago when an enzyme that was needed to convert sugar molecules (glucose) into vitamin C became defunct. This change in the molecules of inheritance (genes) of our ancestors had no immediate disadvantage since, for thousands of generations,

60

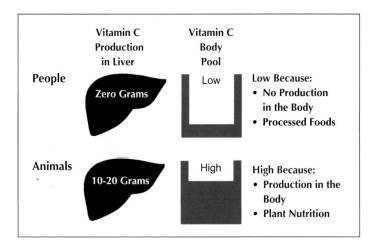

they relied primarily on plant nutrition, such as cereals, fruits and others, that provided the daily minimum of vitamins for them. The nutritional habits and dietary intake of vitamins by humans have changed considerably in this century. Today, most people do not receive sufficient amounts of vitamins in their diets. Still worse, food processing, long-term storage and overcooking destroy most vitamins in food. The consequences are summarized in the picture above.

The single most important difference between the metabolism of human beings and most other living species is the dramatic difference in the body pool of vitamin C. The body reservoir of vitamin C in people is, on average, 10-100 times lower than the vitamin C levels in animals.

## How Does Vitamin C Prevent Atherosclerosis?

Vitamin C contributes in many different ways to the prevention of cardiovascular disease. It is an important antioxidant, and it serves as a cofactor for many biochemical reactions in the body's cells. The most important function of vitamin C in preventing heart attacks and strokes is its ability to increase the production of collagen, elastin and other reinforcement molecules in the body. These biological reinforcement rods constitute the connective tissue, which comprises approximately 50% of all proteins in our bodies. Collagen has the same structural stability function for our bodies as iron reinforcement rods have for a skyscraper building. Increased production of collagen means improved stability for the 60,000-mile-long pipeline of our arteries, veins and capillaries.

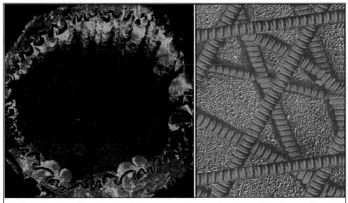

*Left: The cross-section of an artery (magnified). Collagen and other connective tissue (white structures) provide basic stability to blood vessel walls.*

*Right: Individual collagen molecules under high magnification. Each of these fibers is stronger than an iron wire of comparable width.*

The close connection between vitamin C deficiency and the instability of body tissue was established long ago. The following page is taken from the world-famous textbook *Biochemistry* by Professor Lubert Stryer of Stanford University.

# Defective Collagen Hydroxylation Is One of the Biochemical Problems in Scurvy

*"The importance of the hydroxylation of collagen becomes evident in scurvy. A vivid description of this disease was given by Jacques Cartier in 1536 when it afflicted his men as they were exploring the Saint Lawrence River:*

*'Some did lose all their strength and could not stand on their feet...others also had all their skins spotted with spots of blood of a purple color: then did it ascend up to their ankles, knees, thighs, shoulders, arms and necks. Their mouths became stinking, their gums so rotten, that all the flesh did fall off, even to the roots of the teeth, which did also almost all fall out.'*

*The means of preventing scurvy was succinctly stated by James Lind, a Scottish physician, in 1753: 'Experience indeed sufficiently shows that as greens or fresh vegetables with ripe fruits, are the best remedies for it, so they prove the most effectual preservatives against it.' Lind urged the inclusion of lemon juice in the diet of sailors. His advice was adopted by the British navy some 40 years later.*

*Scurvy is caused by a dietary deficiency of ascorbic acid (vitamin C). Primates and guinea pigs have lost the ability to synthesize ascorbic acid, and they must acquire it from their diets. Ascorbic acid, an effective reducing agent, maintains prolyl hydroxylase in an active form, probably by keeping its iron atom in the reduced ferrous state. Collagen synthesized in the absence of ascorbic acid is insufficiently hydroxylated and, hence, has a lower melting temperature. The abnormal collagen cannot properly form fibers and, thus, causes the skin lesions and blood vessel fragility that are so prominent in scurvy."*

From *Biochemistry* by Lubert Stryer

While the vitamin C-collagen connection has been firmly established, the paramount importance of this connection for heart disease has apparently been overlooked or neglected.

# Atherosclerosis Is an Early Form of Scurvy

While these facts have been known for centuries, they still are not applied in medicine today. The next graphic summarizes the fact that the main cause of heart attacks and strokes is a scurvy-like condition of the artery wall.

**Left Column A:** Optimum intake of vitamin C leads to the optimum production and function of collagen molecules. A stable blood vessel wall does not allow atherosclerotic deposits to develop. The optimum availability of vitamin C in their bodies is the main reason why animals don't get heart attacks.

**Right Column C:** The right column of this graphic summarizes the events in scurvy. The total depletion of the body's vitamin C reserves, as they occurred in sailors of earlier centuries, leads to a gradual breakdown of the body's connective tissue, including the blood vessel walls. Thousands of sailors died within a few months from hemorrhagic blood loss through leaky blood vessel walls.

**Center Column B:** Atherosclerosis and cardiovascular disease occur exactly between these two conditions. The average diet contains enough vitamin C to prevent open scurvy, but not enough to guarantee stable, reinforced artery walls. As a consequence, millions of tiny cracks and lesions develop along the artery walls. Subsequently, cholesterol, lipoproteins and other blood risk factors enter the damaged artery walls in order to repair these lesions. With chronically low vitamin intake, however, this repair process continues over decades. Over many years, this repair overcompensates, or overshoots, and atherosclerotic deposits develop. Deposits in the arteries of the heart eventually lead to heart attack; deposits in the arteries of the brain eventually lead to stroke.

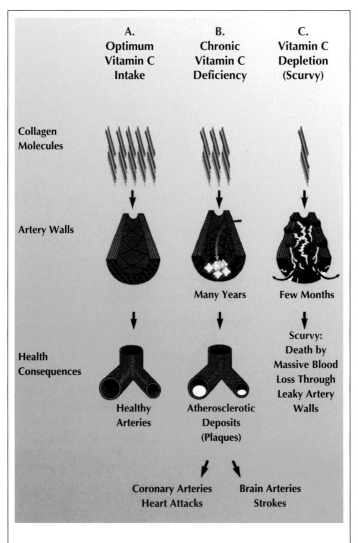

*The scurvy-cardiovascular disease connection*
*The connection between cardiovascular disease, vitamin C deficiency and scurvy is of such fundamental importance to our health that this graphic should become an essential part of health education in schools around the world.*

# Vitamin C Deficiency Causes Atherosclerosis — The Proof

It is possible to prove that insufficient dietary intake of vitamin C alone, without any other factors involved, directly *causes* atherosclerosis and cardiovascular disease. To prove this, we conducted an animal experiment with guinea pigs, which are exceptions in the animal world because they share with humans the inability to produce their own vitamin C. Two groups of guinea pigs received exactly the same daily amounts of cholesterol, fats, proteins, sugars, salt and all other ingredients in their diet with one exception — vitamin C. Group B received 60 mg of vitamin C per day in their diet, compared to human body weight. This amount was chosen to meet the official recommended daily allowance (RDA) for humans in the United States. In contrast, Group A received 5,000 mg of vitamin C per day, compared to human body weight.

These pictures document the changes in the artery walls in these two groups after only five weeks. The first picture shows the differences in the arteries of the two groups. The vitamin C-deficient animals of Group B developed atherosclerotic deposits (white areas), particularly in the areas close to the heart (right side of picture). The aortas of the animals in Group A remained healthy and did not show any deposits. The following pictures show the same artery walls examined under a microscope. The artery sections from animals with high vitamin C intake (Picture 1) show an intact cell barrier between the bloodstream and artery wall. The almost parallel alignment of the collagen molecules in the artery wall makes stability visible. In contrast, the arteries of the vitamin C-deficient animals (Picture 2) lost the protection (defective barrier cell lining) and stability (fragmented collagen structure) of their arteries. For comparison, a picture of the coronary arteries from a patient with coronary artery disease is included (Picture 3).

*Note: In principle, animal experiments should be kept to an absolute minimum. They are only justified when human lives can be saved with the knowledge that results from these experiments. This was the case with the experiment described, which brought proof to millions of people of the value of vitamin C in the prevention of heart attacks.*

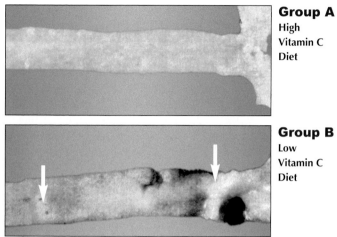

**Group A**
High
Vitamin C
Diet

**Group B**
Low
Vitamin C
Diet

*The main arteries (aortas) of guinea pigs on a high vitamin C diet (**Group A**) and a low vitamin C diet (**Group B**). The white areas in the bottom picture (arrows) are atherosclerotic deposits. These deposits are not the result of a high-fat diet, but of the body's response to the artery wall structure weakened by long-term vitamin-deficiency (magnification below).*

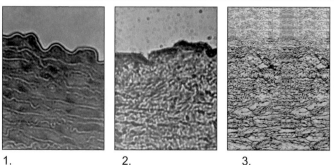

1.   2.   3.

*A view inside three different artery walls under the microscope:*
*1. Guinea pig on a high vitamin C diet*
*2. Guinea pig on a low vitamin C diet*
*3. For comparison: Coronary artery of a patient who died from a heart attack. Note the similarity between the arteries in Picture 2 and Picture 3.*

# Repeating Evolution: Dramatic Confirmation of the Vitamin C-Heart Disease Connection

The final proof for the vitamin C-cardiovascular disease connection was published by a research team from the University of North Carolina, Chapel Hill in the *Proceedings of the National Academy of Sciences* in early 2000. Six years after we received our first patents for the natural prevention and reversal of cardiovascular disease, these researchers confirmed our discovery in a convincing way.

The researchers examined the arteries of normal mice and found that they did not develop atherosclerosis. This was not surprising, since mice normally produce high amounts of vitamin C and cardiovascular disease is, therefore, unknown in normal mice. Then, they experimentally shut down one gene (gulono-lactone-oxidase, GLO) in certain mice. This gene is responsible for converting sugar (glucose) into vitamin C in the livers of mice. Consequently, the mutant mice were no longer able to produce vitamin C in their bodies. With this experiment, the researchers duplicated exactly the situation of human beings: we lack the very same GLO gene and are, therefore, unable to produce vitamin C in our livers.

The decisive question was what would happen to those mutant mice when they — in addition to lacking endogenous vitamin C production in their bodies — received too little vitamin C in their diets? Would their artery walls develop lesions and cracks? Would their cholesterol levels rise in an effort by their bodies to repair this artery wall weakness?

The answer to these questions is "yes." The connective tissue structure (collagen and elastin) of the artery walls of the vitamin C-deficient mice weakened. The cross-section under the microscope strikingly resembles our findings in the experiments on the previous page. Moreover, the vitamin C-deficient mice had significantly higher cholesterol levels. This experiment not only confirmed my discoveries in a dramatic way, but it also

68

terminated any speculation as to whether cholesterol is the cause or the consequence of cardiovascular disease.

This experiment in which only one factor was genetically modified — vitamin C production — confirmed that:

- Vitamin C deficiency is a primary cause of heart disease!

-  High cholesterol is *not the cause of heart disease*, but the *consequence*!

- Cholesterol lowering, without correcting underlying vitamin deficiency, should be considered medical malpractice!

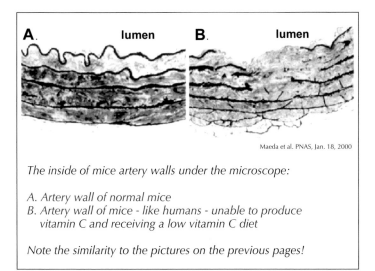

Maeda et al. PNAS, Jan. 18, 2000

*The inside of mice artery walls under the microscope:*

*A. Artery wall of normal mice*
*B. Artery wall of mice - like humans - unable to produce vitamin C and receiving a low vitamin C diet*

*Note the similarity to the pictures on the previous pages!*

69

# A New Understanding of the Nature of Heart Disease

The previous experiment underlines our modern definition of cardiovascular disease as a vitamin deficiency condition. This new understanding is summarized on the opposite page:

1. **Lesions:** The main cause of cardiovascular disease is the instability and dysfunction of the blood vessel wall caused by chronic vitamin deficiency. This leads to millions of small lesions and cracks in the artery wall, particularly in the coronary arteries. The coronary arteries are mechanically the most stressed arteries because they are squeezed flat from the pumping action of the heart more than 100,000 times per day, which is similar to a garden hose being stepped on.

2. **Beginning Repair:** Repair of the artery walls becomes necessary. Cholesterol and other repair factors are produced at an increased rate in the liver and transported in the bloodstream to the artery walls, which they enter in order to mend and repair the damage. Because the coronary arteries sustain the most damage, they require the most intensive repair.

3. **Ongoing Repair:** With continued vitamin deficiency over many years, the repair process in the artery walls overcompensates. Atherosclerotic plaques form predominantly at those locations in the cardiovascular system needing the most intensive repair: the coronary arteries. This is why infarctions occur primarily at this very same location and why the most frequent cardiovascular events are infarctions of the heart, not infarctions of the nose or ears.

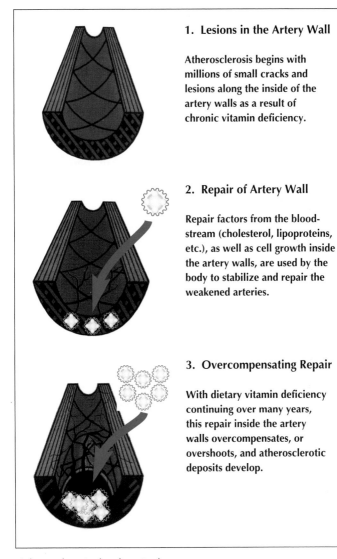

### 1. Lesions in the Artery Wall

Atherosclerosis begins with millions of small cracks and lesions along the inside of the artery walls as a result of chronic vitamin deficiency.

### 2. Repair of Artery Wall

Repair factors from the blood-stream (cholesterol, lipoproteins, etc.), as well as cell growth inside the artery walls, are used by the body to stabilize and repair the weakened arteries.

### 3. Overcompensating Repair

With dietary vitamin deficiency continuing over many years, this repair inside the artery walls overcompensates, or overshoots, and atherosclerotic deposits develop.

*Atherosclerosis develops in three steps.*

# The Natural Reversal of Cardiovascular Disease

The basis for the reversal of atherosclerosis is the initiation of a healing process in the artery wall that has been weakened by chronic vitamin deficiency. Besides vitamin C, which stimulates production of collagen molecules, other constituents of Dr. Rath's Cellular Health recommendations are also essential for this healing process. The graphic on the adjacent page summarizes the protective functions of this essential nutrient program.

In the middle of the graphic is a microscopic cross-section of the atherosclerotic deposit of a human coronary artery. The red area above the plaque represents the area where the blood normally flows. The lipoproteins (fat molecules) in the center of the deposits are stained black with a specific staining technique. Two of these lipoprotein (a) molecules (one lipoprotein (a) and one LDL molecule) among the thousands in this plaque are schematically magnified. These lipoproteins have been deposited inside the artery wall for many years.

Around the core of the plaque, a local "tumor" forms from muscle cells typical in the artery wall. This muscle cell tumor is another way in which the body stabilizes the vitamin-deprived artery wall. The deposit of lipoproteins from the bloodstream and the muscle cell tumor in the artery wall are the most important factors that determine the size of the plaque and, thereby, the progression of coronary heart disease. Any therapy that is able to reverse these two mechanisms of atherosclerosis must also reverse coronary heart disease itself. The nutrients in Dr. Rath's Cellular Health recommendations synergistically affect both mechanisms in the following ways:

1. **Stability of the artery wall through optimum collagen production:** The collagen molecules in our bodies are proteins composed of amino acids. Collagen molecules differ from all other proteins in the body in that they make particular use of the amino acids lysine and proline. We already

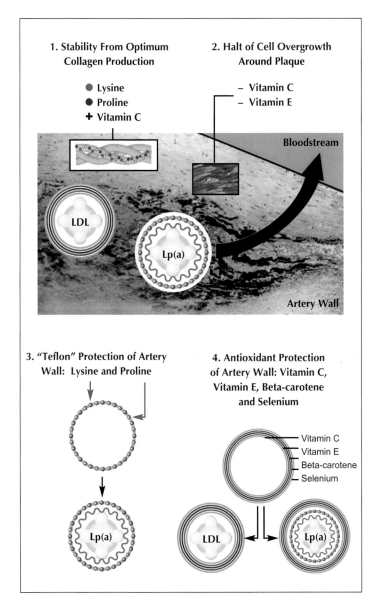

*How atherosclerosis is reversed in a natural way*

know that vitamin C stimulates the production of collagen in the cells of the artery wall. An optimum supply of lysine, proline and vitamin C is a decisive factor in the optimum regeneration of the connective tissue in the artery walls and, therefore, the natural healing of cardiovascular disease.

2. **Decrease of the smooth muscle cell tumor in the artery wall:** With an optimum supply of essential nutrients, the smooth muscle cells of the artery wall produce sufficient amounts of functional collagen, thereby guaranteeing optimum stability of the wall. In contrast, vitamin deficiency leads to the production of faulty and dysfunctional collagen molecules by the arterial muscle cells. Moreover, these smooth muscle cells multiply to form an atherosclerotic tumor. My colleague Dr. Aleksandra Niedzwiecki and her research team investigated this mechanism in detail. They found that vitamin C, in particular, can inhibit the growth of the atherosclerotic "tumor." In the meantime, other studies have shown that vitamin E also has this effect.

3. **"Teflon" protection of the artery wall and reversal of fatty deposits in the artery wall:** Lipoproteins are the transport molecules by which cholesterol and other fat molecules circulate in the blood and attach to the artery wall. For many years, it has been thought that the primary transport molecule responsible for the deposit of fat in the artery walls is LDL (low-density lipoprotein or "bad cholesterol"). Today, we know that the most dangerous fat transport molecules are not LDL molecules, but a variant called lipoprotein (a). The letter (a) could stand for "adhesive," as it characterizes an additional sticky protein that surrounds LDL molecules. By means of this sticky protein, the lipoprotein (a) molecules accumulate inside the artery walls. Thus, it is not the cholesterol or LDL cholesterol level that determines the risk for cardiovascular disease, it is the amount of lipoprotein (a) molecules. In the next chapter, I will discuss this new risk factor in detail.

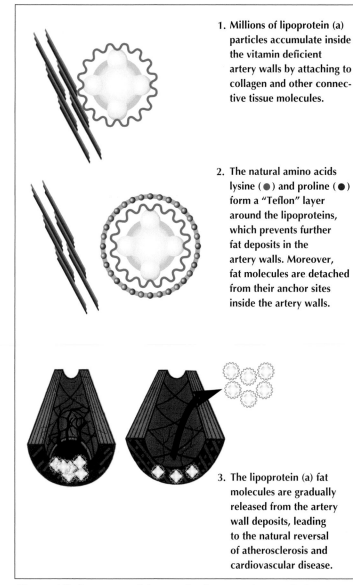

1. Millions of lipoprotein (a) particles accumulate inside the vitamin deficient artery walls by attaching to collagen and other connective tissue molecules.

2. The natural amino acids lysine ( ● ) and proline ( ● ) form a "Teflon" layer around the lipoproteins, which prevents further fat deposits in the artery walls. Moreover, fat molecules are detached from their anchor sites inside the artery walls.

3. The lipoprotein (a) fat molecules are gradually released from the artery wall deposits, leading to the natural reversal of atherosclerosis and cardiovascular disease.

*The world's first patented therapy for the natural reversal of atherosclerotic deposits*

The primary therapeutic aim for preventing fatty deposits in the artery wall is, therefore, to neutralize the stickiness of the lipoprotein molecules and prevent their attachment to the inside of the artery walls. This can be achieved by means of "Teflon" substances for the artery walls. The first generation of these Teflon agents has been identified. They are the natural amino acids lysine and proline. They form a protective layer around the lipoprotein (a) molecules, which has a twofold effect: preventing the deposit of more fat molecules in the artery wall and releasing lipoprotein molecules that have already been deposited inside the artery walls. Releasing fat molecules from the atherosclerotic deposits leads to a natural reversal of cardiovascular disease. Molecule by molecule is released from the atherosclerotic plaques into the bloodstream and transported to the liver, where these molecules are burned. It is important to understand that this is a natural process, and the complications that frequently accompany angioplasty and other mechanical procedures do not occur.

4. **Antioxidant protection in the bloodstream and artery walls:** An additional mechanism accelerating the development of atherosclerosis, heart attacks and strokes is biological oxidation. Free radicals, aggressive molecules found in cigarette smoke, car exhaust and smog, damage the lipoproteins in the bloodstream and the tissue of the artery walls. By doing so, they further increase the size of atherosclerotic plaques. Vitamin C, vitamin E, beta-carotene and other components of Dr. Rath's Cellular Health recommendations belong to the strongest group of natural antioxidants and protect the cardiovascular system from oxidative damage.

The reversal of fatty deposits in the artery wall is a process common in nature. Bears and other hibernators, for example, use it regularly. During several months of winter sleep (hibernation), these animals do not eat and, therefore, get no vitamins from the diet. Moreover, during hibernation, the vitamin C production in their bodies decreases to a minimum. As a consequence, fat molecules and other factors in their blood are deposited in the artery walls and lead to a thickening of these walls. In the spring, after these animals rise from hibernation, their vitamin supply increases dramatically from their diets and their bodies' vitamin production. With this increased vitamin supply, the fatty deposits in the artery walls of these animals gradually reverse, and the artery walls retain their natural stability and function.

The solution to the puzzle of human cardiovascular disease is another striking example of how a close look at nature can help us to find solutions to human diseases.

| Current Conventional "Repair" Medicine | Future Cellular Medicine |
|---|---|

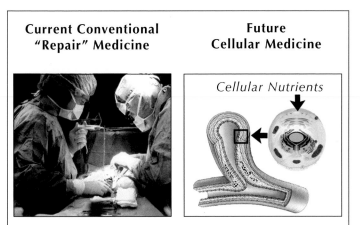

*Cellular Nutrients*

| *Conventional Medicine: Until today, bypass surgery and other mechanical procedures have been the method of choice to treat cardiovascular disease.* | *Cellular Medicine: From now on — and for all future generations — the understanding of the cellular origin of this disease will allow the natural prevention, treatment and, eventually, eradication of it.* |
|---|---|

# Notes

# 3

# High Cholesterol Levels and Other Secondary Risk Factors for Cardiovascular Disease

Dr. Rath's Cellular Health Recommendations for Prevention and Adjunct Therapy

- Cholesterol Is Only a Secondary Risk Factor

- Dr. Rath's Cellular Health Recommendations Help Patients With Elevated Cholesterol Levels

- Clinical Studies With Dr. Rath's Cellular Health Recommendations Document Their Effectiveness in Lowering Blood Risk Factors

- The Cholesterol - Heart Disease Fallacy

# Cholesterol Is Only a Secondary Risk Factor

**Worldwide, hundreds of millions of people** have elevated blood levels of cholesterol, triglycerides, LDL (low-density lipoproteins), lipoprotein (a) and other risk factors. However, cholesterol and all other blood risk factors are considered only "secondary" risk factors because they can only cause damage if the the blood vessel wall is already weakened by vitamin deficiencies. Thus, elevated blood levels of cholesterol and other blood risk factors are not the *cause* of cardiovascular disease — they are the *consequence* of the ongoing vascular disease.

**Conventional medicine,** based on pharmaceutical drugs, is limited to treating the symptoms of cardiovascular disease while ignoring the root cause — blood vessel weakness. Marketing campaigns for cholesterol-lowering drugs simply proclaim cholesterol as the "scapegoat." The latest type of these drugs (statins), which blocks the synthesis of cholesterol is being used by millions of people in the hope for treatment. However, the underlying weakness of the blood vessel wall continues untreated. According to the January 3, 1996 edition of the *Journal of the American Medical Association (JAMA),* statins are known to cause cancer and other severe side effects, and "should be avoided whenever possible."

**Modern Cellular Medicine** provides a new understanding about the factors causing the rise of cholesterol and other secondary risk factors, as well as  their natural prevention. Cholesterol, triglycerides, low-density lipoproteins (LDL), lipoprotein (a) and other metabolic products are ideal repair factors, and their blood levels increase in response to a structural weakening of the artery walls. A chronic weakness of the blood vessel walls increases the demand and, thereby, the production rate of these repair molecules in the liver. An increased production of cholesterol and other repair factors in the liver increases the levels of these molecules in the bloodstream and, over time, renders them risk factors for cardiovascular disease. Thus, the primary measure for lowering cholesterol and other secondary

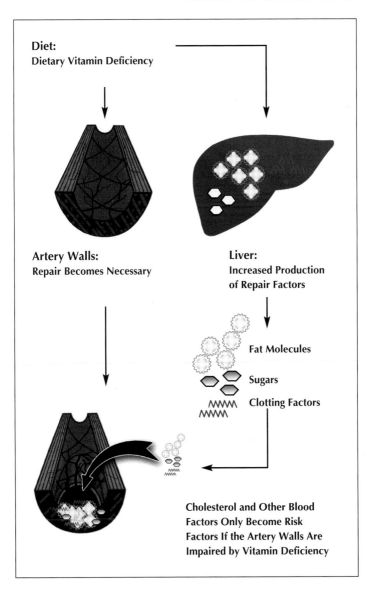

*Elevated cholesterol levels are not the cause, but the consequence of cardiovascular disease.*

risk factors in the bloodstream is to stabilize the artery walls and, thereby, decrease the metabolic demand for increased production of these risk factors in the liver. Therefore, it is not surprising that Dr. Rath's Cellular Health recommendations help to stabilize the artery walls and, at the same time, help to decrease blood levels of cholesterol and other risk factors naturally.

Cellular Medicine helps to expand the understanding about the different factors influencing one's personal risk factor profile. Your basic levels of cholesterol and other blood risk factors are genetically determined and cannot be changed. The two factors you can influence to lower your risk are diet and — above all — intake of specific essential nutrients that regulate cellular metabolism.

**Scientific research and clinical studies** have already documented the particular value of vitamin C, vitamin B3 (nicotinate), vitamin B5 (pantothenate), vitamin E and carnitine, as well as other components of Dr. Rath's Cellular Health recommendations, for lowering elevated cholesterol levels and other secondary risk factors in the blood.

**Dr. Rath's Cellular Health recommendations** comprise a selection of vitamins and other essential nutrients that help to normalize elevated levels of secondary risk factors. These essential nutrients lower the production rate of cholesterol and other repair molecules in the liver and, at the same time, contribute to the repair of the artery walls.

**My recommendations** for patients with elevated cholesterol and other secondary risk factors: lowering cholesterol without first stabilizing the artery walls is an insufficient and ill-fated cardiovascular therapy. Start as early as possible to increase the stability of your artery walls by following the recommendations in this book. As a consequence, blood levels of cholesterol and other risk factors will generally normalize. If you are on cholesterol or lipid-lowering medications, I encourage you to discontinue their use as soon as possible.

# How Dr. Rath's Cellular Health Recommendations Can Help Patients With Elevated Cholesterol Levels

The following section presents letters from patients with cholesterol and other lipid disorders who have been helped by my Cellular Health recommendations. Please share this important information with friends and colleagues to enable them to lower their cholesterol levels in a natural way and to stop taking harmful cholesterol medication.

---

**What You Should Do**

1. **Clear your mind of the belief that cholesterol causes heart disease.**

2. **Stabilize your artery walls with Dr. Rath's Cellular Health recommendations.**

3. **Eat more cereals, vegetables and other fiber-rich foods to "flush out" abundant cholesterol from your body naturally.**

4. **Stop taking cholesterol-lowering medication!**

---

In most people who start following my recommendations, the blood levels of cholesterol and other risk factors in the blood soon decrease. We already know the reason for this effect; this essential nutrient program reduces the production rate of cholesterol and other secondary risk factors in the liver and, thereby, must lead to lower blood levels of this risk factor.

Interestingly, some patients report a transitory rise in cholesterol levels when they start taking vitamins. Because the rise in blood cholesterol levels is not the result of increased cholesterol production, it has to come from other sources — primarily atherosclerotic deposits in the artery walls. This important

83

mechanism was first described by Dr. Constance Spittle in the medical journal *The Lancet* in 1972. She reported that vitamin supplementation in patients with existing cardiovascular disease frequently led to a temporary increase of cholesterol levels in the blood. In contrast, the cholesterol levels of healthy test persons did not rise with vitamin supplementation.

The temporary rise in cholesterol is an additional sign of the healing process in the artery walls and the decreasing of fatty deposits. The mechanism described here is, of course, not only valid for cholesterol, but also for triglycerides, LDL, lipoprotein (a) and other secondary risk factors, which have accumulated over decades inside the artery walls and have been slowly released into the bloodstream.

**My recommendations in this case:** Should your cholesterol levels rise when you start following these recommendations, it can indicate the reversal of existing deposits in your artery walls. You should continue the vitamin program until, after several months, the blood level of cholesterol decreases below the initial values. A diet high in soluble fiber (e.g. oat bran, cereals and pectins) can further decrease cholesterol and other secondary risk factors in the blood.

The following letters document the rise and subsequent decrease of cholesterol in patients following Dr. Rath's Cellular Health recommendations:

*Dear Dr. Rath:*

*I had started taking a fiber product in February of 1994.* **My cholesterol continued to climb from 280 to over 320 until May of 1994, when I began to follow your recommended vitamin program.**

**My cholesterol has dropped to 180 and my ratio of HDL to LDL is normal, as is my triglyceride level.** *Most important, however, my lipoprotein (a) dropped from 15 to 1! I will continue your program forever.*

*Thank you, Dr. Rath, for your work with natural therapies as a means for decreasing the risk of heart disease.*

*With much gratitude,*
*M.R.*

---

*Dear Dr. Rath:*

*I am 45 years old, and since December of last year I have been on your program of essential nutrients. I also take a fiber formula.* **Last April, my cholesterol level was 259. This April, after only 4 months on this program, my cholesterol dropped to 175!**

*Dr. Rath, I truly want to thank you for helping me to be healthier and live a much fuller life.*

*Sincerely,*
*M.W.*

Dear Dr. Rath:

Heart disease is hereditary within my family, and my father had his first heart attack in his early 30s. I had my cholesterol checked at age 19 only to find out that **I had a cholesterol level of 392 mg/dl**. My physician did not want to place me on medication at that time, so I just watched my diet and increased my exercise. Well, as time passed, my cholesterol remained elevated, and my physician felt medication was necessary. I refused to begin medication and continued with diet and exercise.

At age 26, I had my cholesterol tested before I began your vitamin program, and my lab test showed a reading of 384. I immediately began following your program, with a fiber drink, and my level dropped 120 points within a 6-10 week period. **Over a four-month period, my LDL went from 308 down to 205.** This is a program that I personally follow, and continue to have positive results.

I recommend it to my family and friends.

Sincerely,
C.C.

*Dear Dr. Rath:*

*I began taking a fiber formula two years ago in September. My total cholesterol was around 177 at that time. Within 90 days, I lost 20 pounds and my total cholesterol dropped to 154.*

*In November last year, I started with your vitamin program. An insurance physical that was done in February of this year showed a total cholesterol (CHOL) level of 191, a triglyceride level of 244, a LDL/HDL ratio of 4.09 and a CHOL/HDL ratio of 6.8, all which were elevated. Again, note that this was in February.*

*A cholesterol screening was done in March and again in June. Both showed a total cholesterol level of 134.* ***A lipid profile that was done in July showed a total cholesterol level of 135, a triglyceride level of 180, a LDL/HDL ratio of 1.47 and CHOL/LDL ratio down to 3.16 from 6.8.***

*Your cardiovascular health program is working!*

*Sincerely,*
*L.M.*

# Clinical Studies With Dr. Rath's Cellular Health Recommendations Document Their Effectiveness in Lowering Blood Risk Factors

The effect of vitamin C on the blood levels of cholesterol and other blood fats has been documented in numerous clinical studies. More than 40 of these studies have been evaluated by Dr. Harrie Hemilä of the University of Helsinki, Finland. In patients with high initial cholesterol values (above 270 mg per deciliter), vitamin C supplementation was able to decrease cholesterol levels up to 20%. In contrast, patients with low and medium initial values of cholesterol showed only a slight cholesterol-lowering effect or the levels stayed the same.

In a study sponsored by the American Heart Association, Dr. B. Sokoloff showed that two to three grams of vitamin C per day could lower triglyceride blood levels on average by 50% - 70%. It was shown that vitamin C increased the production of enzymes (lipases) able to degrade triglycerides and lower triglyceride levels.

Dr. Jacques and his colleagues showed that people taking 300 mg of vitamin C per day also had much higher HDL blood levels than people taking less than 120 mg per day. This is particularly important since HDL (high-density lipoproteins) are fat-transporting molecules that can pick up cholesterol and other fats from the artery walls and carry them back to the liver for removal. This is yet another way vitamin C can help reduce atherosclerotic deposits and reverse cardiovascular disease. Dr. W.J. Hermann and his colleagues reported that vitamin E supplementation also increases HDL blood levels.

Further clinical studies show that other components of Dr. Rath's Cellular Health recommendations work synergistically with vitamin C in lowering cholesterol and other blood fats. These components include vitamin B3 (nicotinic acid), vitamin B5 (pantothenate), vitamin E, carnitine and other essential nutrients. This synergistic effect is an important advantage over megadose intake of individual vitamins.

| Cellular Nutrients Tested | Reference |
|---|---|
| Vitamin C | Ginter, Harwood and Hemilä |
| Vitamin B3 | Altschul, Carlson and Guraker |
| Vitamin B5 | Avogaro, Cherchi and Gaddi |
| Vitamin E | Beamish and Hermann |
| Carnitine | Opie |

# Lipoprotein (a) — A Secondary Risk Factor Ten Times More Dangerous Than Cholesterol

Now I would like to introduce you to a particularly important secondary risk factor, lipoprotein (a). The genuine function of lipoprotein (a) is very useful; it fulfills a variety of repair functions, for example, during wound healing. However, if the artery wall is destabilized by a long-term vitamin deficiency, lipoprotein (a) turns into a risk factor 10 times more dangerous than cholesterol. Let's take a closer look at how lipoprotein (a) molecules differ from other fat molecules.

**Cholesterol and triglycerides** do not float in the blood in the way that fat floats in soup. Thousands of cholesterol molecules are packed together with other fat molecules in tiny round globules called lipoproteins. Millions of these fat-transporting vehicles circulate in our bodies at any given time. The best known among these lipoproteins are high-density lipoproteins (HDL, or "good cholesterol") and low-density lipoproteins (LDL, or "bad cholesterol").

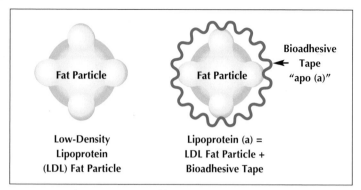

*Comparison between LDL and lipoprotein (a)*

**LDL cholesterol:** Most of the cholesterol molecules in the blood are transported in millions of LDL particles. By carrying cholesterol and other fat molecules to our bodies' cells, LDL is a very useful transport vehicle for supplying nutrients to these cells. LDL has been named "bad cholesterol" because, until recently, researchers believed that LDL was primarily responsible for the fatty deposits in the artery walls. This understanding is now out of date.

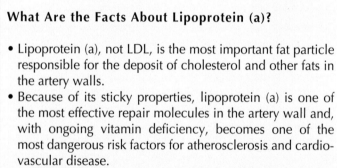

### What Are the Facts About Lipoprotein (a)?

- Lipoprotein (a), not LDL, is the most important fat particle responsible for the deposit of cholesterol and other fats in the artery walls.
- Because of its sticky properties, lipoprotein (a) is one of the most effective repair molecules in the artery wall and, with ongoing vitamin deficiency, becomes one of the most dangerous risk factors for atherosclerosis and cardiovascular disease.
- A re-evaluation of the Framingham Heart Study, the largest cardiovascular risk factor study ever conducted, showed that lipoprotein (a) is a tenfold greater risk factor for heart disease than cholesterol or LDL cholesterol.

**Lipoprotein (a)** is an LDL particle with an additional adhesive protein surrounding it. This biological "adhesive tape" is named apoprotein (a) or, apo (a). The letter (a) could, in fact, stand for "adhesive." The adhesive apo (a) makes the lipoprotein (a) fat globule one of the stickiest particles in our bodies.

---

**In a Vitamin-Deficient Body, Lipoprotein (a) Becomes the Most Important Secondary Risk Factor for:**

- Coronary Heart Disease and Heart Attacks
- Cerebrovascular Disease and Strokes
- Restenosis (Clogging) After Coronary Angioplasty
- Clogging of Bypass Grafts After Coronary Bypass Surgery

---

Together with my colleagues at Hamburg University, I conducted the most comprehensive studies on lipoprotein (a) in the artery wall. These studies showed that the atherosclerotic lesions in human arteries are largely composed of lipoprotein (a) rather than LDL molecules. Moreover, the size of the atherosclerotic lesions paralleled the amount of lipoprotein (a) particles deposited in the arteries. In the meantime, these findings have been confirmed in a series of additional clinical studies.

Lipoprotein (a) blood levels vary greatly between one individual and another. What do we know about the factors influencing the lipoprotein (a) levels in the blood? Lipoprotein (a) levels are primarily determined by inheritance. Special diets do not influence lipoprotein (a) blood levels. Moreover, none of the presently available lipid-lowering prescription drugs lower lipoprotein (a) blood levels.

The only substances that have, thus far, been shown to lower lipoprotein (a) levels are vitamins. Professor Carlson showed that two to four grams of vitamin B3 (nicotinic acid) a day could lower lipoprotein (a) levels up to 36%. Because high levels of nicotinic acid can cause skin rashes, you are advised to increase the daily intake of nicotinic acid gradually. Our own research has shown that vitamin C alone or in combination with lower dosages of nicotinic acid may also have a lowering effect on the production of lipoproteins, and thereby, lower lipoprotein blood levels. Together with the "Teflon" agents lysine and proline, these two vitamins can considerably decrease the cardiovascular risk associated with lipoprotein (a) levels.

---

**Therapeutic Approaches to Reduce the Risk From Lipoprotein (a)**

1. Lowering of Lipoprotein (a) Blood Levels
   – Vitamin B3 (Nicotinate)
   – Vitamin C

2. Decreasing Stickiness of Lipoprotein (a)
   – Lysine
   – Proline

---

Lipoprotein (a) is a particularly interesting molecule because of its inverse relationship to vitamin C. The following discovery triggered my interest in vitamin research: lipoprotein (a) molecules are primarily found in humans and in a few animal species unable to produce vitamin C. In contrast, animals able to produce optimum amounts of vitamin C do not need lipoprotein (a) in any significant amount. Lipoprotein (a) molecules apparently compensate for many properties of vitamin C, such as wound healing and blood vessel repair. In 1990, I published the details of this important discovery in the *Proceedings of the National Academy of Sciences* and cited Dr. Linus Pauling as co-author of this publication.

# The Cholesterol – Heart Disease Fallacy

While reading this section, you may have asked yourself the questions: "But what about cholesterol? Are those reports about cholesterol only media hype?" Unfortunately, this is the case. Here are some of the sobering facts:

The leading medical speculation about the origin of cardiovascular disease is as follows: high levels of cholesterol and risk factors in the blood damage the blood vessel walls and lead to atherosclerotic deposits. According to this hypothesis, lowering cholesterol is the primary measure to prevent cardiovascular disease. Tens of millions of people worldwide are currently taking cholesterol-lowering drugs with the expectation that they will help fight cardiovascular disease. The marketing propaganda behind these cholesterol-lowering drugs is worthy of a closer look.

In the 70s, the World Health Organization (WHO) conducted an international study to determine whether cholesterol-lowering drugs could decrease the risk for heart attacks. Thousands of study participants received the cholesterol-lowering drug "Clofibrate." This study could not be completed because those people who took the cholesterol-lowering drug experienced too many side effects. Thus, in the interest of the health and lives of the study participants, this cholesterol-lowering drug study had to be called off.

In the early 80s, a large-scale study in more than 3,800 American men made headline news. This study tested whether the cholesterol-lowering drug "Cholestyramine" could lower the risk for heart attacks. One study group took up to 24 grams (24,000 mg) of Cholestyramine every day over several years. The control group of this study took the same amount of  a placebo (ineffective control substance). The results of this study were that in the cholesterol-lowering drug group, the same number of people died as in the control group. Particularly frequent among those patients taking this cholesterol-lowering

93

drug were accidents and suicides. Irrespective of these facts, those interested in marketing the drug decided to promote this study as a success. The fact that in the drug group there were slightly fewer incidences of heart attacks was marketed as a confirmation of the cholesterol-heart attack hypothesis. Few people bothered with the actual death figures of this study.

In the late 80s, a new group of cholesterol-lowering drugs was introduced, which was shown to decrease the production of cholesterol in the body. Soon thereafter, it was determined that these drugs not only lowered the production of cholesterol in the body, but also lowered the manufacture of other essential substances, for example, ubiquinone (coenzyme Q-10). Karl Folkers, MD, of the University of Texas at Austin, rang the alarm bells in the *Proceedings of the National Academy of Sciences*. Dr. Folkers reported that patients with existing heart failure who took these new cholesterol-lowering drugs could experience life-threatening deterioration of their heart function.

A giant blow for the cholesterol-lowering drug industry came on January 6, 1996. On this day, the *Journal of the American Medical Association* published an article entitled "Carcinogenicity of Cholesterol-Lowering Drugs." Dr. Thomas Newman and Dr. Stephen Hulley, of the University of California, San Francisco Medical School, showed that most of the cholesterol-lowering drugs on the market were known to cause cancer in test animals at levels currently prescribed to hundreds of thousands of people. The results from this article were so alarming that the authors raised the legitimate question: "How could it be that the regulatory agency, the U.S. Food and Drug Administration (FDA), allowed these drugs to be sold to millions of people?" The answer given by the authors of this study: "The pharmaceutical companies manufacturing these drugs downplayed the importance of these side effects and, thereby, removed any obstacles for their approval."

The publication of the first edition of this book in 1993 explained for the first time to a broad audience that animals don't get heart attacks because they produce enough vitamin C, not because they have low cholesterol levels. Heart attacks are the primary result of vitamin deficiencies — not elevated cholesterol. It was immediately clear that cholesterol-lowering drugs, beta-blockers, calcium antagonists and many other pharmaceuticals would eventually be replaced by essential nutrients in eliminating cardiovascular disease.

The time needed to reach this goal would be dependent on one single factor only: how fast the knowledge about the connection between scurvy and cardiovascular disease could be spread. The manufacturers of cardiovascular drugs knew that they would lose a drug market worth trillions of dollars over time. This multi-trillion dollar global market of symptom-oriented drugs will inevitably collapse once millions of people learn that vitamins and other essential nutrients are the answer to the cardiovascular disease epidemic.

This is the background of why the pharmaceutical industry is spending hundreds of millions of dollars fighting the natural Cellular Medicine alternative and advertising drugs that do not cure, but cause new diseases such as cancer.

# Why Bears Are Not Extinct

If anyone among my readers still thinks that cholesterol may cause heart attacks, I would like to share the following facts: Bears, and millions of other hibernating animals, have average cholesterol levels of over 400 mg per deciliter. If cholesterol were indeed the culprit causing heart attacks and strokes, bears and other hibernating animals would have long ago become extinct as a result of heart attacks. The reason why bears are still among us is simple — they produce high amounts of vitamin C in their bodies, which stabilize their artery walls so they are unaffected by cholesterol.

The fact that bears are not extinct proves:

1. Elevated cholesterol blood levels are not the primary cause of atherosclerosis, heart attacks and strokes.
2. Achieving and maintaining stability of the artery walls through an optimum vitamin supply is more important than lowering cholesterol and other risk factors in the bloodstream.
3. Cholesterol and other repair factors in the bloodstream can only become risk factors if the artery walls are weakened by chronic vitamin deficiency.

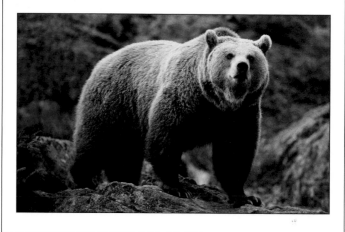

# Cellular Health Recommendations for Patients With High Cholesterol and Other Metabolic Disorders

**In addition, to my Basic Cellular Health recommendations (page 25), I recommend that patients with elevated cholesterol levels and other metabolic disorders take the following cellular bioenergy factors in higher dosages:**

- **Vitamin C:** for the protection and natural healing of the artery walls, lowering increased production of cholesterol and other secondary risk factors in the liver and reducing elevated blood levels of these secondary risk factors

- **Vitamin E:** for antioxidant protection of blood fats and millions of cells

- **Vitamin B1:** for optimizing cellular metabolism and, particularly, for the delivery of bioenergy

- **Vitamin B2:** for optimizing cellular metabolism and, particularly, for the delivery of bioenergy

- **Vitamin B3:** for lowering the elevated production of cholesterol and lipoproteins in the liver

- **Vitamin B5:** for the structural component of the central metabolic molecule of cells (coenzyme A) and optimal metabolic burning of fat molecules

- **Vitamin B6, Biotin and Folic Acid:** for counteracting increased levels of the risk factor *homocysteine and* optimizing the metabolism of cells

- **Carnitine:** for optimizing cellular metabolism of fats and lowering triglyceride levels

97

# Notes

# High Blood Pressure

Dr. Rath's Cellular Health Recommendations
for Prevention and Adjunct Therapy

- The Facts About High Blood Pressure

- Dr. Rath's Cellular Health Recommendations:
  - Documented Health Benefits in Patients
  - Documented Health Benefits by Clinical Studies

- Scientific Background Information

# The Facts About High Blood Pressure

**Worldwide, several hundred million people suffer from high blood pressure.** Of all cardiovascular health conditions, this is the single largest epidemic. The epidemic spread of this disease is largely due to the fact that, until now, the causes of high blood pressure have been insufficiently, or not at all, understood.

**Conventional medicine** concedes that the causes of high blood pressure are unknown in over 90% of patients. The frequent medical diagnosis "essential hypertension" was established to describe high blood pressure conditions in which the causes remain unknown. Conventional, pharmaceutical-oriented medicine is confined to treating the symptoms of this disease. Beta-blockers, diuretics and other high blood pressure medications artificially lower the blood pressure (symptom-oriented approach) without correcting the primary underlying problem — a "spasm" of the blood vessel wall.

**Modern Cellular Medicine** provides a breakthrough in our understanding of the causes, prevention and adjunct treatment of high blood pressure. The main cause of high blood pressure is a chronic deficiency of essential nutrients in millions of artery wall cells. Among other functions, these cells are responsible for the availability of "relaxing factors" (nitric oxide), which decrease vascular wall tension and keep the blood pressure in normal range. The natural amino acid arginine, vitamin C and other components of Dr. Rath's Cellular Health recommendations contribute to the optimum availability of these artery wall relaxing factors. In contrast, chronic deficiency of these essential nutrients can result in spasms and a thickening of the blood vessel walls, which can eventually elevate blood pressure.

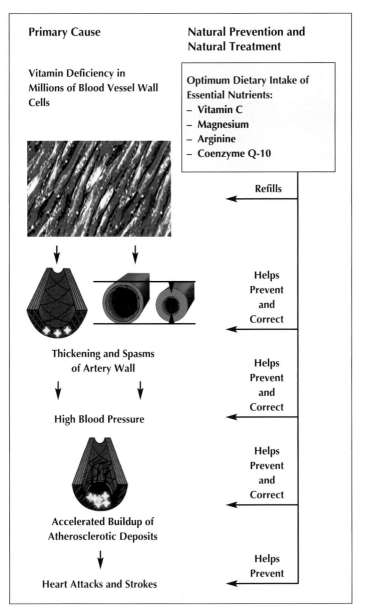

*The causes, prevention and adjunct treatment of high blood pressure*

**Scientific research and clinical studies** have documented the value of vitamin C, magnesium, coenzyme Q-10, arginine and other essential nutrients in helping to normalize high blood pressure conditions. Dr. Rath's Cellular Health recommendations comprise select essential nutrients that are needed for the optimum functioning of vascular wall cells and, thereby, contribute to preventing high blood pressure and helping reverse existing high blood pressure conditions.

**My recommendations** for high blood pressure patients: Start immediately with these Cellular Health recommendations and inform your doctor about it. Follow this program in addition to using your regular medication. Do not stop or change your regular medication without consulting your doctor.

**Prevention is better than treatment.** The success of Dr. Rath's Cellular Health recommendations in patients with high blood pressure is based on the fact that the millions of artery wall cells are supplied with "cell fuel" for optimum function. A natural cardiovascular program that contributes to correcting high blood pressure conditions is, of course, your best choice in preventing the development of high blood pressure in the first place.

# How Dr. Rath's Cellular Health Recommendations Can Help Patients With High Blood Pressure

The following section presents a selection of letters from patients with high blood pressure who are following Dr. Rath's Cellular Health recommendations. With the help of this book, millions of high blood pressure patients around the world can now also take advantage of this natural medical breakthrough.

---

*Dear Dr. Rath:*

*About 8 weeks ago, I was introduced to a fiber product for the reduction of my cholesterol, which had reached 260 in spite of my efforts to get it down. After being on that product about 2 and a half weeks, I realized that my blood pressure was going up. **I have been on blood pressure medication for essential hypertension since my teen years.** I supposed that it was due to the energy I was feeling from the fiber formula.*

*Then I heard that your essential nutrient program could lower blood pressure. I immediately started on your program. **Within two weeks, my blood pressure had gone from 145/150 over 90/96 to 130/82 - sometimes a bit higher if I am really busy!** I also noticed a lessening of a feeling of chest pressure, and I could breathe deeper.*

*Sincerely,*
*S.S.*

---

Dear Dr. Rath:

I am a 53-year-old man, and my blood pressure was being controlled by blood pressure medication. **I had been taking blood
pressure medication of various types for 10 years.**

**After 4 months on your cardiovascular vitamin program, I went
off all blood pressure medication, and my blood pressure was
checked every two weeks.** My blood pressure has now been normal for 6 weeks, with your cardiovascular health program.
I had noticed some angina prior to this program, and those symptoms have also been eliminated.

Sincerely,
J.L.

---

Dear Dr. Rath:

**I have been following your Cellular Health recommendations for
five months. In the meantime, my doctor reduced my blood
pressure medication by half** so I can honestly say I'm now taking
half the medication I was five months ago. I am maintaining a
blood pressure average of 120/78. Thrilled? You'd better believe
it! Next goal: no medication at all. Thank you again.

Sincerely,
L.M.

*Dear Dr. Rath:*

*I am a 52-year-old male with a high blood pressure problem that spans 25 years. I've been through six different physicians, and I've lost count of the different blood pressure medications that have been prescribed for me. The best that any doctor was able to reduce my blood pressure to was an average of 135/95 for the last five or six years, with a combination of prescription medication.*

*I began following your vitamin program last December. My blood pressure dropped to an average of 124/82 by the first week of January, and I experienced a greater feeling of energy and well-being. That occurred despite no change in diet or lifestyle.* **My doctor reduced one of my blood pressure medications by half, and my blood pressure still dropped over the next few months to an average of 122/80.**

*The third week of May last year, it dropped to 120/64. So far, that level seems to be the start of a trend, so I'll have to visit my doctor again for a further reduction in medication.*

*I am now absolutely convinced that your recommendations did really help to lower my blood pressure and all I can say is a big "Thank You."*

*Sincerely,*
*L.M.*

# Background Information on Dr. Rath's Cellular Health Recommendations in High Blood Pressure

This page summarizes in more detail the mechanisms by which Dr. Rath's Cellular Health recommendations help patients to normalize high blood pressure. The following therapeutic mechanisms have been identified for one or more of the ingredients of this vitamin program:

**Arginine**, the natural amino acid, splits off an artery wall "relaxing factor," a small molecule called nitric oxide. Nitric oxide increases the elasticity of the artery walls and helps to normalize high blood pressure.

**Vitamin C** increases the production of prostacycline, a small molecule that not only relaxes the blood vessel walls, but also keeps blood viscosity at optimum levels.

**Magnesium,** "nature's calcium antagonist," is essential for an optimum mineral balance in the blood vessel wall cells. Optimum mineral balance is a precondition for the relaxation of the artery walls.

**Lysine and proline** help protect the artery walls and prevent the development of atherosclerotic deposits. This important mechanism was discussed in Chapters Two and Three of this book in detail. Since atherosclerosis is intertwined with high blood pressure, these ingredients are also essential for preventing and correcting this health condition.

All these nutrients are components of my Cellular Health recommendations.

# A Clinical Study With Dr. Rath's Cellular Health Recommendations in High Blood Pressure

Dr. Rath's Cellular Health recommendations were tested in a clinical pilot study with 15 patients suffering from severe hypertension. The patients, ranging in age between 32-69, participated in the study for a period of 32 weeks. They followed my Cellular Health recommendations in addition to taking their prescribed high blood pressure medications.

Each patient's blood pressure was measured bi-weekly for the duration of the study. At the beginning of the study, all patients had elevated systolic and diastolic blood pressure readings. The average systolic blood pressure reading was 167, and the average diastolic blood pressure reading was 97.

After 32 weeks of following my Cellular Health recommendations, the blood pressure of all patients improved. At the end of the study, patients had an average systolic blood pressure reading of 142 and an average diastolic blood pressure reading of 83. These readings were 16% and 15% lower, respectively, than the measurements taken at the beginning of the study. These results were achieved without any side effects.

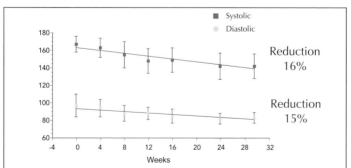

*In patients following Dr. Rath's Cellular Health recommendations, diastolic and systolic blood pressure levels were lowered by 16% (systolic value) and 15% (diastolic value), respectively — without any side effects.*

107

# Other Clinical Studies With Cellular Nutrients in High Blood Pressure

Various clinical studies show that different components of my Cellular Health recommendations are able to lower high blood pressure. The following table summarizes some of the most important studies:

| Cellular Nutrients Tested | Blood Pressure Lowered | Reference |
|---|---|---|
| Vitamin C | 5%–10% | McCarron |
| Coenzyme Q-10 | 10%–15% | Digiesi |
| Magnesium | 10%–15% | Turlapaty and Widman |
| Arginine | More than 10% | Korbut |

It is important to note that in all these studies the natural components helped to normalize blood pressure, but did not cause a too-low blood pressure situation. This is another advantage compared to conventional medication, where overdosing frequently leads to decreased blood circulation, dizziness and other health problems.

# Specific Cellular Health Recommendations for Patients With High Blood Pressure

In addition to the Cellular Health recommendations found on page 25, I recommend that patients with elevated blood pressure take the following nutrients in higher dosages:

**Vitamin C:** decreases tension of the artery wall, increases supply of relaxing factors and lowers elevated blood pressure

**Vitamin E:** provides antioxidant protection and protection of cell membranes and blood components

**Arginine:** improves production of "relaxing factors," decreases tension of the artery walls and lowers elevated blood pressure

**Magnesium:** optimizes cellular metabolism of minerals, decreases tension of the blood vessel walls and lowers elevated blood pressure

**Calcium:** optimizes mineral metabolism, decreases tension of the artery walls and lowers elevated blood pressure

**Bioflavonoids:** catalysts, which among others, improve the efficacy of vitamin C

# Notes

**5**

# Heart Failure

Dr. Rath's Cellular Health Recommendations
for Prevention and Adjunct Therapy

- **The Facts About Heart Failure**

- **The Fatal Consequences of Incomplete Treatment
  of Heart Failure**

- **Dr. Rath's Cellular Health Recommendations:**
  - **Documented Health Benefits in Patients**
  - **Documented Health Benefits by Clinical Studies**

# The Facts About Heart Failure

**Tens of millions of people** worldwide suffer from heart failure, which results in shortness of breath, edema and fatigue. The number of heart failure patients has tripled over the last few decades. The epidemic spread of this disease is largely due to the fact that, until now, the causes of heart failure have been insufficiently, or not at all, understood. In some cases, heart failure is the result of a heart attack; in most cases, however, such as with cardiomyopathies, heart failure develops without any prior cardiac event.

**Conventional medicine** is largely confined to treating the symptoms of heart failure. Diuretic drugs are given to flush out the water that is retained in body tissues because of the weak pumping function of the heart. However, they also flush out water-soluble micronutrients, thereby causing additional health problems. The still insufficient understanding of the causes of heart failure explains the unfavorable prognosis of this disease. Five years after a heart failure condition is diagnosed, only 50% of the patients are still alive. For many patients with heart failure, a heart transplant operation is the last resort. Most heart failure patients, however, die without ever having the option of such an operation.

**Cellular Medicine** provides a breakthrough in the understanding of the causes, prevention and adjunct treatment of heart failure. The primary cause of heart failure is a deficiency of vitamins and other essential nutrients providing bioenergy to the millions of heart muscle cells. These cells are responsible for the contraction of the heart muscle and for the optimum pumping of blood into circulation. Deficiencies of vitamins and other essential nutrients impair the pumping performance of the heart, resulting in shortness of breath, edema and fatigue.

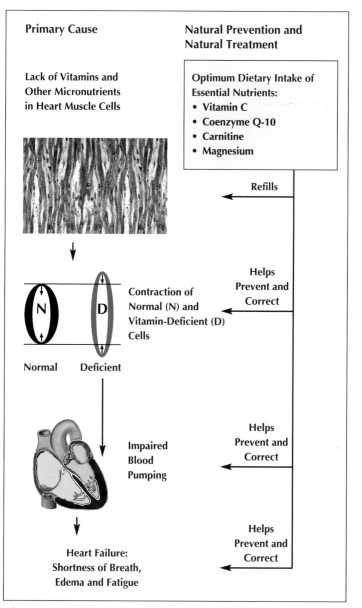

The causes, prevention and adjunct treatment of heart failure

113

# The Fatal Consequences of Incomplete Treatment of Heart Failure

For decades, the focus of conventional medicine on diuretics and other symptom-oriented pharmaceutical drugs has prevented the discovery of the true cause of heart failure. Moreover, the conventional treatment of heart failure patients shows how the lack of understanding about the root cause of a disease leads to a vicious cycle in which therapeutic measures worsen the health problem.

Today, we know that the chronic deficiency of essential cellular nutrients in heart muscle cells impairs the pumping function of the heart. This leads to impaired blood circulation in different organs of the body. For example, the kidneys remove excess water by filtering it from the blood into the urine. With impaired blood flow through the kidneys, water is retained in tissues and causes swelling (edema) of the legs, lungs and other parts of the body.

In order to eliminate edema, doctors prescribe diuretic medications. This measure starts a vicious cycle in the conventional therapy of heart failure. Diuretics remove water-soluble vitamins, such as vitamins C and B, and important minerals and trace elements from the body. Since vitamin deficiency is already the main cause of heart failure, diuretic medications further aggravate the disease.

Now we understand why the prognosis of heart failure is so unfavorable. The future therapy of heart failure is straightforward: the supplementation of vitamins and other essential cellular nutrients. If water has accumulated in a patient's body, diuretics should be given. Irrespective of that, the daily supplementation of essential cellular nutrients must become an essential part of any heart failure therapy.

As a heart failure patient, you should talk with your doctor about these findings. A responsible physician will support this essential nutrient program.

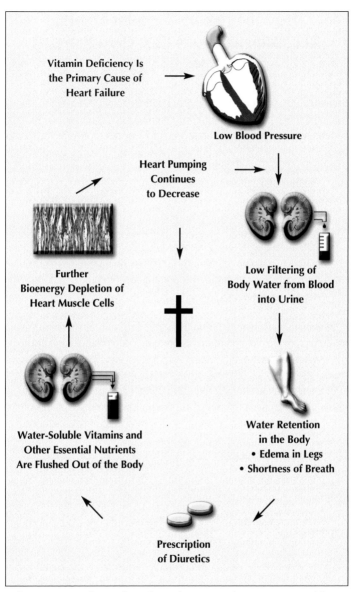

Vitamin Deficiency Is the Primary Cause of Heart Failure

Low Blood Pressure

Heart Pumping Continues to Decrease

Further Bioenergy Depletion of Heart Muscle Cells

Low Filtering of Body Water from Blood into Urine

Water-Soluble Vitamins and Other Essential Nutrients Are Flushed Out of the Body

Water Retention in the Body
• Edema in Legs
• Shortness of Breath

Prescription of Diuretics

*The vicious cycle resulting from the incomplete treatment of heart failure is the reason for the fatal prognosis of this disease.*

# How Dr. Rath's Cellular Health Recommendations Can Help Patients With Heart Failure

**Scientific research and clinical studies** have already documented the particular value of carnitine, coenzyme Q-10 and other essential nutrients. These components of Dr. Rath's Cellular Health recommendations help improve the function of millions of heart muscle cells, the pumping function of the heart itself and, thereby, the quality of life of heart failure patients.

**My recommendations** for heart failure patients: Start immediately following these recommendations and inform your doctor about it. Follow them in addition to using your regular medication. Do not stop or alter your regular medication without consulting your doctor.

**Prevention is better than treatment.** The success of Dr. Rath's Cellular Health recommendations in heart failure patients is based on the optimum supply of "cell fuel" to the millions of heart muscle cells. A natural health program that is able to correct cardiovascular health conditions such as heart failure is your best choice in preventing these problems from developing in the first place.

**Documented Success:** The following section presents a selection of letters from heart failure patients who are following Dr. Rath's Cellular Health recommendations. With the help of this book, millions of these patients around the world can also now take advantage of this natural medicine breakthrough.

Please share this information with anyone you know who suffers from shortness of breath, edema or chronic fatigue. You may help save a life.

*Dear Dr. Rath:*

*Our sister-in-law was diagnosed with **congestive heart failure.** She was told by her physician to go home and get her affairs in order, sell her home and prepare to move into a nursing home because she was only going to get worse and wouldn't be able to care for herself. **Her chest was full of fluids, she had to sleep sitting up, she was too weak to walk and her legs were swelling.***

***She started your Cellular Health recommendations late in February, and in three weeks, she was feeling well enough to go out for dinner, get her hair done and put her house on the market.***

*She has since moved into a nice retirement home, and she goes everywhere the bus goes. She is so grateful that she has been given her life back and never wants to be without your vitamin program.*

*Sincerely,*
*R.A.*

---

*Dear Dr. Rath:*

*I am happy to report that your Cellular Health recommendations have improved my life. **Now I can climb the stairs readily without shortness of breath. I can also resume hiking for 3-4 miles a day without feeling tired and exhausted.** I do have an energetic outlook towards life, and I'm sure it's due to your cardiovascular vitamin recommendations.*

*Thank you very much for all the research you have done and that you continue to do for people with circulatory problems.*

*Sincerely,*
*A.G.*

*Dear Dr. Rath:*

*I am a 46-year-old female. Six years ago, I had a severe reaction to a prescription medication. The ultimate result of that was that I had severe congestive heart failure. I was diagnosed as having valvular regurgitation of the mitral, tricuspid and pulmonary valves (leaking of heart valves), as well as mitral valve prolapse. My clinical symptoms were extreme fatigue, shortness of breath, edema, tachycardia and pulmonary edema.*

*Since following your Cellular Health recommendations, I am now taking only a beta-blocker for medication. All others have been stopped. My symptoms are now only occasional fatigue. **I do not have severe shortness of breath, I can carry on a conversation without sounding out of breath and I am able to exercise on a daily basis. There is no edema, tachycardia (rapid heartbeat), or pulmonary congestion.***

*Your Cellular Health recommendations have given me an entirely new outlook on the future, where at one time I did not feel that there would be a future.*

*Sincerely,*
*J.T.*

---

*Dear Dr. Rath:*

*For three months now, I have been following your cardiovascular vitamin program.*

*I just returned from my usual 4-mile walk at a brisk pace, up two small hills, and around the neighborhood with no discomfort at all. **For the first time, I am absolutely free of distress.***

*Best wishes,*
*J.H.*

*Dear Dr. Rath:*

*I am a 36-year-old female.* **Since my late 20s, I have experienced episodes of arrhythmia and shortness of breath. I also had begun to have edema in my ankles.** *My heart rate was usually between 88 and 98. My blood pressure averaged 140/86.*

*Being a nurse, I knew to discontinue salt and caffeine. Upon doing so, the symptoms improved for a while. The past few years, however, I was beginning to require medication and was about to get further medical attention for my cardiac changes when I was introduced to your cardiovascular vitamin program last February.*

**Now, four months later, I no longer require medication for the edema, nor do I have any arrhythmia, shortness of breath, or palpitations.** *I have always continued my aerobic exercise, which I was beginning to have difficulty in sustaining. However, my stamina has improved tremendously over these past few months.*

*My heart rate now averages 78 and my blood pressure was 112/60 last week. Thank you!*

*Sincerely and in good health,*
*V.G.*

*Dear Dr. Rath:*

*I started your Cellular Health nutrient program the same week I read your book "Why Animals Don't Get Heart Attacks, But People Do."*

*Unlike many things in this world, your presentations are so basic and simple that everyone can understand the principles involved. My hope is that everyone in this country and the world will receive your message and have the same good results that I did.*

***I have eliminated my diuretic medications completely and cut my blood pressure medication in half since I started following your vitamin program.*** *I'm now reading 120/78 at age 69, and I feel great.*

*My doctor was surprised and pleased, and told me to continue the preventative health care path that started with your program. This program is unique and your patent on the technology to reverse heart disease without surgery is, as you say, like patenting nature — and it works.*

*Thank you so much for your work and for sharing your research with so many people. The world will be a happier place because of you.*

*Sincerely,*
*B.B.*

*Dear Dr. Rath:*

**Since 1989, I have been suffering from congestive heart failure**
*and to this day, I am still following the originally prescribed med-
ication with good results. However, I noticed that I was unable to
perform any small effort or even walk a couple of blocks without
suffering chest pain, and I had to alleviate its intensity by ingesting
a tablet. It was usual for me to take 3-5 tablets every 24 hours,
since the pain would surface sometimes for no apparent reason.*

**I started following your vitamin program in January. After only
four months on your vitamin program, I not only rarely use the
nitroglycerin tablets, but I am walking 1.1 miles every morning
at a brisk pace, with no shortness of breath and no chest pain.**

*Please keep in mind that my hometown's altitude is 5,280 feet
above sea level. I'll be 75 next October. Thought you'd be interested to read about this.*

*Yours truly,*
*F.W.*

# Dr. Rath's Cellular Health Recommendations Can Render Heart Transplants Redundant

After visiting with a heart failure patient and his cardiologist, I documented the following report about the health improvement of this patient. From now on, heart failure patients around the world can benefit from Cellular Health recommendations that provides essential bioenergy to heart muscle cells. This case is just one example.

> G.P. is an entrepreneur in his 50s. **Three years ago, his life was changed by a sudden occurrence of heart failure,** a weakness of the heart muscle leading to a decreased pumping function and enlargement of the heart chambers. The patient could no longer fully meet his professional obligations and had to give up all his sports activities. **On some days, he felt so weak that he couldn't climb stairs, and he had to hold his drinking glass with both hands.** Because of the continued weak pumping function of the heart and the unfavorable prognosis of this disease, his cardiologist told him, "I recommend you get a new heart."
>
> At this point, the patient started to follow the vitamin program I developed. His physical strength improved gradually. **Soon, he could again fulfill his professional obligations on a regular basis and was able to enjoy daily bicycle rides. Two months after following my recommendations, his cardiologist noted a decrease in the size of his previously enlarged heart in an echocardiography examination, another sign of a recovering heart muscle.** One month later, the patient was able to take a business trip abroad, and he could attend to his business affairs without any physical limitations.

The health improvement of another heart failure patient, Joey B., was even featured on the "CBS Evening News" in Memphis, Tennessee.

At age 21, Joey suddenly developed a severe form of heart failure and was hospitalized with "cardiomyopathy." Shortly thereafter, she underwent a heart transplant surgery and received a new heart.

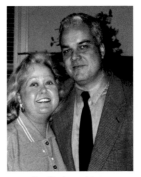

After four years, Joey's new heart had become so weak that her doctors suggested a second heart transplant. At age 25, the flight attendant was scheduled to receive another new heart.

*Dr. Rath and Joey*

At that point in her life, Joey learned about my cellular nutrient program, and she started following it. After six months, her cardiologists reassessed the necessity for the second heart transplant operation. To their astonishment, they found that Joey's heart had recovered so much that there was no need for another heart transplant operation.

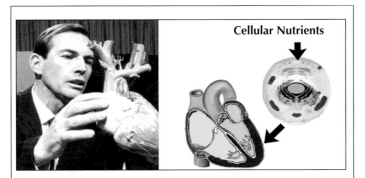

**Cellular Nutrients**

Cellular Bioenergy Instead of Heart Transplant

*No medical procedure was more celebrated than the first heart transplant operation by the South African physician Christian Barnard, M.D. Now, decades later, we understand that the treatment of heart failure is not the replacement of the organ but, instead, the refuelling of bioenergy to millions of heart muscle cells.*

123

# Clinical Studies in Heart Failure Patients With Dr. Rath's Cellular Health Recommendations

## A. Improved Heart Pumping Function

The Cellular Health recommendations described here were tested in a clinical study with heart failure patients. In this pilot study, six patients ages 40-66 were included. At the beginning of the study, the heart performance of these patients was measured by echocardiography (ultrasound examination of the heart). This test measures how much blood the heart pumps into circulation with every heartbeat (ejection fraction). In addition, the physical performance of the patients was assessed with a treadmill test.

Then, the patients followed my Cellular Health recommendations *in addition to* using their regular medication. After two months on this program, echocardiography and treadmill tests were conducted again. The results showed that with this nutritional supplement program, the ejection fraction and physical performance increased on average by 20%. Thus, by following my Cellular Health recommendations, heart function in these patients improved beyond any result obtained by prescription drugs.

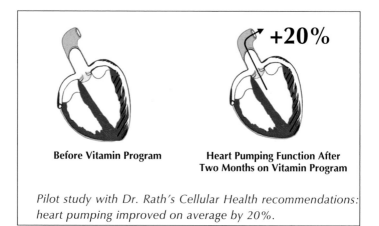

**Before Vitamin Program**

**Heart Pumping Function After Two Months on Vitamin Program**

*Pilot study with Dr. Rath's Cellular Health recommendations: heart pumping improved on average by 20%.*

## B. Improved Quality of Life

In another clinical pilot study, 10 patients with heart failure followed my Cellular Health recommendations for six months. The regular (pharmaceutical) drugs they had been taking before the study were continued during this time.

The severity of their heart failure symptoms (edema, shortness of breath, dyspnea, etc.) was assessed at the beginning of this study by the standard grading system of the New York Heart Association (NYHA):

1. Any physical activity possible without symptoms
2. Moderate physical activity causes symptoms
3. Slightest physical activity causes symptoms
4. Symptoms present at rest

Considering the fact that conventional medicine has no root cause treatment for heart failure, the results of this clinical study with cellular nutrients were remarkable: eight out of 10 patients improved their health condition by one or more grades on the NYHA scale. After six months, half of the patients could lead normal lives again without any discomfort.

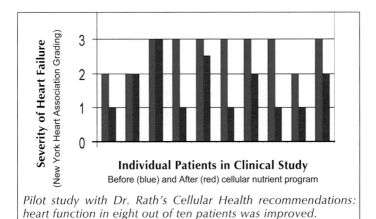

*Pilot study with Dr. Rath's Cellular Health recommendations: heart function in eight out of ten patients was improved.*

125

Heart failure affects the entire body, and patients suffer from a variety of health problems that affect their quality of life. In this study, we also assessed the effect of these Cellular Health recommendations on specific symptoms of heart failure, such as irregular heartbeat (tachycardia), shortness of breath (dyspnea) and inability to perform daily work (severe fatigue).

After six months with Dr. Rath's Cellular Health recommendations, the following improvements were documented and compared to the start of the study when the patients were on prescription drugs only:

- Irregular heartbeat disappeared in all eight patients who initially suffered from this condition (100% improved).
- Severe fatigue was eliminated in all nine patients who initially suffered from this condition (100% improved).
- Shortness of breath was no longer present in five out of seven patients with initial dyspnea (70% improved).

In addition, these health improvements were achieved without any side effects. The results are summarized in the following graph:

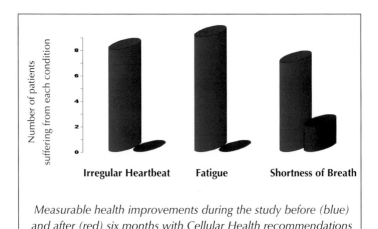

*Measurable health improvements during the study before (blue) and after (red) six months with Cellular Health recommendations*

# Further Clinical Studies With Selected Cellular Nutrients in Heart Failure

In numerous independent clinical studies, compounds of my Cellular Health recommendations have been documented to greatly help people with shortness of breath, edema and other heart failure conditions.

---

**Clinically Proven Health Benefits of Essential Nutrients for Heart Failure Patients**

- **Improved Pumping Function of the Heart**
- **Normalization of Enlarged Heart Chambers**
- **Less Shortness of Breath**
- **Less Edema**
- **Improved Physical Performance**
- **Significantly Longer Life Expectancy**

---

**Coenzyme Q-10:**

The most comprehensive clinical studies tested coenzyme Q-10 and carnitine, carrier molecules of bioenergy in the millions of heart muscle cells. For example, Peter Langsjoen, MD and Karl Folkers, MD and their colleagues at the University of Texas at Austin showed that heart failure patients taking coenzyme Q-10 in addition to their regular medication could significantly improve their survival chances. After three years, 75% of those patients who took coenzyme Q-10 in addition to their regular medication were still alive, whereas of those patients who took only their regular medication, only 25% were still alive. In other words, every second patient in this study owed his or her life to coenzyme Q-10 supplementation.

**Thiamine (Vitamin B1):**

In a clinical study published in the *American Journal of Medicine*, Dr. Shimon and his colleagues studied the health benefits of vitamin B1 supplementation in heart failure. Thirty patients with heart failure, receiving diuretic and other conventional

127

drug therapies, were tested over a period of six weeks. The effects of this cellular nutrient on heart function were measured by echocardiography. Vitamin B1 supplementation increased the cardiac pumping function (left ventricular ejection) of the heart failure patients by 22%. Moreover, the improved heart function also had a natural diuretic effect and decreased water retention (edema) in patients.

**Carnitine:**
In a clinical study conducted by Dr. Rizos and published in the *American Heart Journal,* 80 patients with heart failure were studied over a period of three years. Half of the patients received daily carnitine supplementation in addition to conventional therapy, and the other half of the patients received a placebo only.

At the end of the study, in the placebo group 18% of the patients had died from heart failure complications. In contrast, in the carnitine treated group only 3% of the patients had died. This clinical study showed that carnitine can statistically increase the chances of survival in patients with heart failure.

| Cellular Nutrients Tested | Reference |
| --- | --- |
| Coenzyme Q-10 | Folkers and Langsjoen |
| Carnitine | Rizos and Ghidini |
| Vitamin B1 | Shimon |

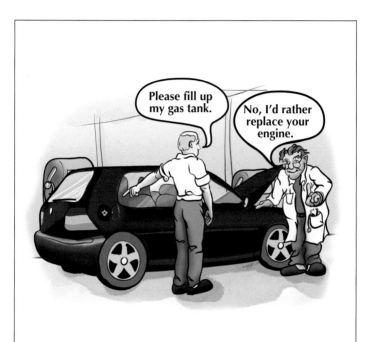

The conventional approach to heart failure is summarized in this cartoon. Treating a heart failure condition with a heart transplant operation is like replacing your car engine when you simply ran out of fuel. Cellular Medicine provides the cellular energy for the "motor" of your body.

# Cellular Health Recommendations for Patients With Heart Failure

**In addition to my Basic Cellular Health recommendations described in Chapter One, I recommend that patients with shortness of breath, edema and chronic fatigue take the following cellular bioenergy factors in higher dosages:**

- **Vitamin C:** supplies energy for the metabolism of each cell and supplies the bioenergy carrier molecules of the vitamin B group with lifesaving bioenergy

- **Vitamin E:** provides antioxidative protection and, especially, protection of the cell membranes

- **Vitamins B1, B2, B3, B5, B6, B12 and Biotin:** bioenergy carriers of cellular metabolism and, particularly, for the heart muscle cells, improved heart function, heart pumping and improved physical endurance

- **Coenzyme Q-10:** the most important element of the "respiratory chain" of each cell; plays a particular role in improved heart muscle function because of the high bioenergy demand of the heart muscle cells

- **Carnitine:** improves supply of bioenergy for the "power plants" (mitochondria) of millions of cells

- **Taurine:** a natural amino acid whose lack in the heart muscle cells is a frequent cause of heart failure

# Notes

# 6

# Irregular Heartbeat
# (Arrhythmia)

Dr. Rath's Cellular Health Recommendations
for Prevention and Adjunct Therapy

- **The Facts About Irregular Heartbeat**

- **Dr. Rath's Cellular Health Recommendations:**
  - **Documented Health Benefits in Patients**
  - **Documented Health Benefits by Clinical Studies**

# The Facts About Irregular Heartbeat

**Worldwide, more than 100 million people** suffer from irregular heartbeat. This condition is caused by a disturbance in the creation or conduction of the electrical impulse responsible for a regular heartbeat. In some cases, these disturbances are caused by a damaged area of the heart muscle, for example, after a heart attack. The textbooks of medicine, however, admit that in most cases the causes of irregular heartbeat remain unknown. It is no wonder that irregular heartbeat conditions are a growing epidemic on a worldwide scale.

**Conventional medicine** has invented its own diagnostic term to cover the fact that it does not know the origin of most arrhythmias. "Paroxysmal arrhythmia" means nothing other than "causes unknown." As a direct consequence, the therapeutic options of conventional medicine are confined to treating the symptoms of irregular heartbeat. Beta-blockers, calcium antagonists and other anti-arrhythmic drugs are given to patients in the hope that they will decrease the incidence of irregular heartbeat. However, the most frequent known side effect of these drugs is an increased risk for new arrhythmias!

Slow forms of arrhythmias with long pauses between heartbeats are dealt with by implanting a pacemaker. In other cases, heart muscle tissue that creates or conducts uncoordinated electrical impulses is cauterized (burned) and eliminated as a focus of the electrical disturbance in the heart muscle. Without an understanding of the primary cause of irregular heartbeat, the therapeutic approaches by conventional medicine are not specific and frequently fail.

**Modern Cellular Medicine** now provides the breakthrough in our understanding of the causes, prevention and adjunct treatment of irregular heartbeat. The most frequent cause of irregular heartbeat is a chronic deficiency of vitamins and other essential nutrients in millions of "electrical" heart muscle cells that generate and conduct the electrical impulse responsible

134

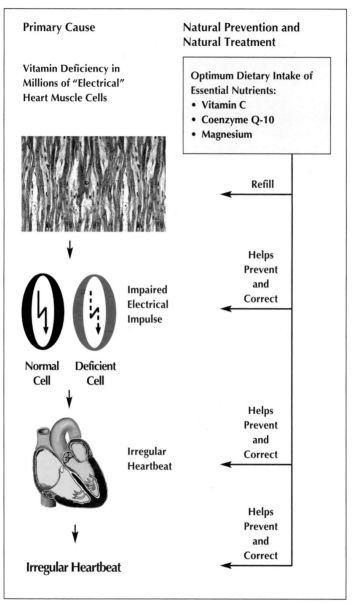

*The causes, prevention and adjunct treatment of irregular heartbeat*

for a normal heartbeat. Long-term deficiencies of essential nutrients in these cells cause or aggravate disturbances in the creation or conduction of the electrical impulses and trigger arrhythmias. The primary method for preventing and correcting irregular heartbeat is an optimum supply of specific vitamins and other cellular nutrients.

**Scientific research and clinical studies** have already documented the value of magnesium, carnitine, coenzyme Q-10 and other important components of my Cellular Health recommendations in helping to normalize different forms of irregular heartbeat and improve the quality of life for patients.

**My recommendations** for patients with irregular heartbeat: Start as soon as possible with this vitamin program and inform your doctor about it. Take these essential nutrients in addition to your regular medication. Do not stop or alter your regular medication on your own. Any changes in anti-arrhythmic medication can have serious consequences for your heartbeat and should be done only in consultation with your doctor.

**Prevention is better than treatment.** A natural cardiovascular program, which helps to correct severe health conditions such as irregular heartbeat is, of course, your best choice for preventing irregular heartbeat in the first place.

# How Dr. Rath's Cellular Health Recommendations Can Help Patients With Irregular Heartbeat

Please share the following letters with anyone you know suffering from irregular heartbeat. By doing so, you may help greatly improve the quality of life of a person or even save a life.

---

*Dear Dr. Rath:*

***Two months ago, I was experiencing loud heartbeats, tachycardia and irregular beating of my heart.*** *I saw my doctor who promptly put me on an anti-arrhythmic drug. I can honestly say the medication did me absolutely no good.*

*Then, I started to follow your vitamin program. What a smart decision that was!* ***Within a few days, the tachycardia stopped and I've not experienced any loud or irregular heartbeats.*** *It's like a miracle. It must be the combination of nutrients in your program because I had been taking coenzyme Q-10 separately from my regular vitamins. I tell everyone I know about the benefits of your program. Because of your research, I'm able to continue working.*

*Sincerely,*
*B.M.*

---

*Dear Dr. Rath:*

*In February, I introduced my 74-year-old grandmother to your cardiovascular vitamin program.* ***Her slow and irregular heartbeat had led her doctor to begin preliminary preparations to install a pacemaker.***

***After about three weeks on your program, her heart action was sufficiently improved to cause the doctor to postpone this procedure.*** *This lady is now a faithful follower of your cardiovascular health program and, although she faces other medical challenges, her heart condition continues to improve and the use of a pacemaker is no longer being considered.*

*Sincerely,*
*K.C.*

---

137

*Dear. Dr. Rath:*

*I am excited to tell you of my experience. I am a 60-year-old female who has fought hypertension for the past 20 years with many different types of medications, which would work for a while, then become ineffective and start giving me problems.*

*In November of 1993, new symptoms began for which I was referred to a cardiologist who determined I was well on my way to a pacemaker. He decided not to treat this aggressively, but instead, through medication. I have avoided surgery. **In February of this year, I began experiencing prolonged bouts of tachycardia and was prescribed new, additional medication.***

*In March, I was introduced to your cardiovascular vitamin program. Although I was skeptical, I decided to give it a try. I've just started my third month on your nutrient program, and I have been able to reduce my blood pressure medication by one-third.*

***The episodes of tachycardia have decreased dramatically, both in intensity and duration. If an episode occurs, it is almost insignificant. At the same time, I have also noted a dramatic effect in that my ankles are no longer swelling at the end of a workday.***

*Following my last lab work, my doctor told me, "Your numbers look like someone half your age." Needless to say, I am a staunch believer in your vitamin program.*

*Sincerely,*
*F.S.*

Dear Dr. Rath:

**I am 54 years of age and have had a very irregular heartbeat for at least 20 years. This was diagnosed as second degree electrical heart block.** I have never taken any medication for this. I have had a stress test done approximately every 2 years and the heart block showed up on the EKG. I was told that as long as my heartbeat was regular when I exercised, I did not need any other treatment.

In June, I even went back to the doctor where I had my last EKG done so there would be a basis for comparison. **The doctor found that there was no longer any arrhythmia. I have enclosed a copy of his report.** I am sure that your cardiovascular vitamin program is responsible for the correction of my irregular heartbeat, as I had not changed my lifestyle in any other respect.

Sincerely,
T.H.

---

Dear Dr. Rath:

**How delightful when, after following your cardiovascular health program for just 2 months, one notices the absence of irregular heartbeats and the freedom to breathe freely.** Confidence is restored as one has increased vigor and endurance. In a word, one spends less time thinking about the heart and more time enjoying life.

Your cardiovascular nutrient program has become the answer for resolving coronary problems. I am happy to have this opportunity of expressing my gratitude for your advanced medical research and for your cardiovascular health program.

Yours sincerely,
J.S.

*Dear Dr. Rath:*

*Thank you for developing your essential nutrient program, which I am currently following.* **Several years ago, I was diagnosed as having Hyperkinetic Heart Syndrome.** *I took medication for a few years, but did not like how I felt — too slowed down and not able to respond quickly to physical exertion.*

**During times of great stress, I would have pounding, irregular, and racing heartbeats at nighttime when I was trying to fall asleep.** *Also, when confronted with a stressful encounter during the day, my heart would immediately jump into a racing, pounding episode. I heard your lecture in May, and I immediately read two of your books.*

**A week later, I began following your cardiovascular vitamin recommendations and within a few days, I was no longer experiencing pounding, irregular, and racing heartbeats at bedtime. Within a week, I noticed that when confronted with a stressful encounter during the day, my heart did not jump into a racing and pounding episode.**

*I have taken vitamins, minerals, and herbal supplements for several years, but have never had this amazing result before now! Thank you so very much!*

*Yours truly,*
*C.M.*

*Dear Dr. Rath:*

*I am a 35-year-old medical professional. One and one-half years ago, due to severe distress in my professional and personal lives, **I suddenly experienced bouts of supraventricular tachycardia (fast heartbeat), which forced me into the emergency room every two months** over a six-month period. My average heart rate would be 230 beats per minute. This condition was life threatening, and after my third episode, I was referred to the chief of cardiology at the largest hospital in town. After a thorough evaluation, it was concluded that I was not suffering from "anxiety," but a primary electrical problem with my heart and the supraventricular tachycardia could occur anytime.*

*Therefore, he recommended a surgical procedure called cardiac ablation. This procedure involved the insertion of catheters into my subclavian and femoral arteries, threading them to the sinus and atrioventricular nodal regions of the heart. A DC current would cauterize certain regions of the heart theorized to be the cause of this aberrant electrical circuit. Although this procedure was definitely indicated, I was too weakened from my recent bout with tachycardia to consider immediate surgery. I therefore resolved to improve my health by strengthening myself nutritionally with vitamins, minerals and herbal and homeopathic formulas.*

*My research led me to your cardiovascular health program. Your formulation was specific to my health needs, and it saved me much time considering I would have purchased many bottles of isolated ingredients that are all found in your program. Therefore, I embarked on a religious program of supplementation of the essential nutrients you recommended. **It has been one and one-half years since my last episode. I have increased energy and little to no chest pain. I look and feel much better.** I attribute my success and health to your program.*

*Sincerely,*
*S.S.*

# A Double-Blind Placebo-Controlled Clinical Study Confirms Dr. Rath's Cellular Health Recommendations Can Reduce Irregular Heartbeat

Until today, conventional medicine did not recognize the basic understanding that irregular heartbeat is caused by a deficiency of bioenergy-carrying nutrients in the heart muscle cells as the underlying mechanism of this disease.

In Eugene Braunwald's *Heart Disease — A Textbook of Cardiovascular Medicine,* the leading textbook of cardiology, we find the remarkable confession of one of the leading conventional cardiologists: "It is important to realize that our present diagnostic tools do not permit the determination of the mechanisms responsible for most arrhythmias."

Considering this dramatic lack of progress after a century of conventional medical research into the causes of irregular heartbeat, the need to solve this puzzle is obvious. It is even more urgent, considering the fact that millions of patients worldwide need no longer suffer from this condition.

With the support of thousands of patients I had already helped with my Cellular Health recommendations, we conducted the first independent clinical study with cellular nutrients in patients with irregular heartbeat. The scientific value and credibility of these study results are beyond any doubt because it was conducted as a so-called "double-blind placebo-controlled" study. This is the same type of study pharmaceutical companies need to conduct in order to get acceptance for their drugs. The complete study can be reviewed on our website www.dr-rath-research.org.

One hundred and thirty-one patients suffering from irregular heartbeat (atrial arrhythmia) were involved in this study. They were divided into two groups. One group followed my cardiovascular nutrient program, and the other group received an ineffective placebo pill. Both groups continued their pharmaceutical drug plan as prescribed by their doctors. The study was conducted over a period of six months.

The results showed that my nutrient program was able to:

1. Decrease the episodes of irregular heartbeat in 30% of the patients.
2. Continuously decrease irregular heartbeat over the duration of the nutrient program.
3. Double the chances of a patient being completely free of irregular heartbeat.

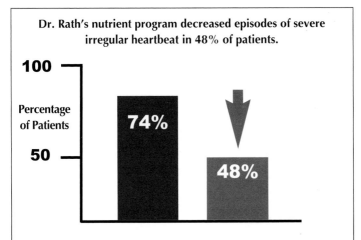

Results of the first double-blind placebo-controlled clinical study testing a natural nutrient program to fight arrhythmia

*Approximately 74% of patients on pharmaceutical drugs only (blue) continued to suffer from frequent episodes of irregular heartbeat. In patients following my nutrient program — in addition to taking their medication — these episodes were stopped in nearly half of the patients (48%), a result that was statistically highly significant (p<0.01).*

Even more important were the additional findings about the benefits of my nutrient program in improving overall physical health, as well as mental health. This data was evaluated using an extensive questionnaire in which patients had to answer specific questions as to their physical and mental health conditions. Each patient had to complete this questionnaire at the beginning and end of the study. This comprehensive data was evaluated using a computer-based grading system to meet international scientific standards. Physical health questions evaluated included, for example, the discomfort during episodes of irregular heartbeat and the patients' ability to conduct their daily work. Mental health questions included the patients' fear of heart dysfunction, as well as related depression.

The results were remarkable. Patients on my cellular nutrient program outperformed the placebo patients approximately four times in physical and mental health improvements.

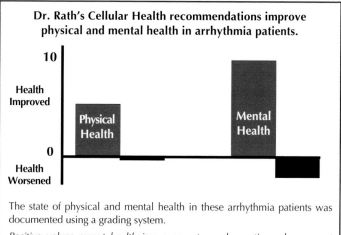

The state of physical and mental health in these arrhythmia patients was documented using a grading system.

*Positive values meant health improvements, and negative values meant health deterioration. Patients following my nutritional recommendations (red column) improved their physical and mental health, compared to patients taking drugs only (black column), whose conditions worsened.*

# Solving the Puzzles of Cardiology

## Why are arrhythmias particularly frequent in young women of childbearing age?

One of the unsolved puzzles of conventional cardiology is the fact that arrhythmias are particularly frequent in young women of childbearing age.

Without understanding the underlying cause of these arrhythmias in young women, they are frequently prescribed anti-arrhythmic drugs with known severe side effects, including the induction of even more episodes of irregular heartbeat.

It is an inexusable failure of conventional cardiology to have neglected for almost a century a thorough investigation of this important health problem affecting the lives of millions of young women.

The scientific breakthrough of Cellular Medicine provides the immediate and obvious answer to this medical puzzle. During her childbearing years, every woman loses a significant amount of blood during the menstrual cycle. It is not only blood that is lost, but also its constituents, including vitamins, minerals and other essential nutrients needed to maintain cellular energy metabolism in the organs.

The "electrical" heart muscle cells responsible for the generation and conduction of the electrical impulse for regular heartbeat are among the first cells affected by this deficiency. Thus, the prevention and treatment of choice for arrhythmias — particularly in young women — is the daily supplementation of essential nutrients.

# Cellular Health Recommendations for Patients With Irregular Heartbeat

**In addition to my Basic Cellular Health recommendations described in Chapter One, I recommend that patients with irregular heartbeat take the following cellular bioenergy factors in higher dosages (compare to heart failure recommendations):**

### Vitamin C:
supplies energy for the metabolism of each cell and supplies the bioenergy carrier molecules of the vitamin B group with lifesaving cellular energy

### Vitamins B1, B2, B3, B5, B6, B12 and Biotin:
bioenergy carriers of cellular metabolism and, particularly, for the "electrical" heart muscle cells responsible for the generation and conduction of the electrical impulse for normal heartbeat

### Coenzyme Q-10:
the most important element of the "respiratory chain" of each cell; it plays a particular role in the energy metabolism of heart muscle cells

### Carnitine:
contributes to the efficient utilization of cellular bioenergy in the "power plants" (mitochondria) of millions of heart muscle cells

### Magnesium and Calcium:
required, together with potassium, for the optimum conduction of electrical impulses during the electrical heartbeat cycle

## Notes

# 7

# Diabetes

**Dr. Rath's Cellular Health Recommendations
for Prevention and Adjunct Therapy**

- The Facts About Adult Onset Diabetes

- How Diabetic Cardiovascular Disease Develops

- Dr. Rath's Cellular Health Recommendations:
  - Documented Health Benefits in Patients
  - Documented Health Benefits by Clinical Studies

# The Facts About Adult Onset Diabetes

**Worldwide, more than 100 million people suffer from diabetes.** Diabetic disorders have a genetic background and are divided into two types: juvenile and adult. Juvenile diabetes is generally caused by a genetic defect that leads to an insufficient production of insulin in the body and requires regular insulin injections to control blood sugar levels. The majority of diabetic patients, however, develop this disease as adults. Adult forms of diabetes also have a genetic background. However, the causes that trigger the outbreak of the disease in these patients at any stage in their adult lives have been unknown. It is, therefore, not surprising that diabetes is yet another disease that is still growing on a global scale.

**Conventional medicine** is confined to treating the symptoms of adult diabetes by lowering elevated blood levels of sugar. However, cardiovascular disease and other diabetic complications occur even in those patients with controlled blood sugar levels. Thus, lowering blood sugar levels is a necessary, but incomplete, treatment of diabetic disorders.

**Modern Cellular Medicine** now provides a breakthrough in our understanding of the causes, prevention and adjunct treatment of adult diabetes. The primary cause of adult onset diabetes is a long-term deficiency of certain vitamins and other essential nutrients in the millions of cells in the pancreas (the organ that produces insulin), the liver and the blood vessel walls, as well as other organs. On the basis of an inherited diabetic disorder, deficiencies of vitamins and other essential nutrients can trigger a diabetic metabolism and the onset of adult diabetes. Conversely, the optimum intake of vitamins and other ingredients in Dr. Rath's Cellular Health recommendations can help prevent the onset of adult diabetes and help correct existing diabetic conditions and its complications.

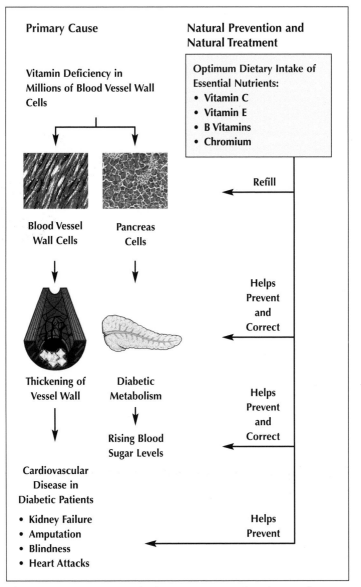

**Primary Cause**

**Natural Prevention and Natural Treatment**

**Vitamin Deficiency in Millions of Blood Vessel Wall Cells**

**Optimum Dietary Intake of Essential Nutrients:**
- **Vitamin C**
- **Vitamin E**
- **B Vitamins**
- **Chromium**

**Blood Vessel Wall Cells**

**Pancreas Cells**

**Refill**

**Thickening of Vessel Wall**

**Diabetic Metabolism**

**Helps Prevent and Correct**

**Rising Blood Sugar Levels**

**Helps Prevent and Correct**

**Cardiovascular Disease in Diabetic Patients**
- **Kidney Failure**
- **Amputation**
- **Blindness**
- **Heart Attacks**

**Helps Prevent**

*The causes, prevention and adjunct treatment of cardiovascular complications in diabetes*

151

**Scientific research and clinical studies** have documented the particular value of vitamin C, vitamin E, certain B vitamins, chromium and other essential nutrients in helping to normalize a diabetic metabolism and prevent cardiovascular disease.

**My recommendations for diabetic patients:** Start immediately with this program of essential nutrients and inform your doctor about it. Take the essential nutrients in addition to your diabetes medication, and do so regularly. High amounts of vitamin C, for example, can spare insulin units, and you should have additional blood sugar controls at the beginning of this vitamin program. Do not stop or change any prescription medication without consulting your doctor.

**Prevention is better than treatment.** The success of my Cellular Health recommendations for diabetic patients is based on the fact that this program eliminates a deficiency of biological fuel in the millions of cells in the pancreas, liver and blood vessel wall. A natural cardiovascular health program that is able to correct severe conditions such as diabetes is, of course, your best choice in preventing diabetes and its cardiovascular complications in the first place.

# Cardiovascular Disease Is the Key Complication for Diabetic Patients

Diabetes is a particularly malicious metabolic disorder. Circulatory problems and clogging can occur in virtually any part of the 60,000-mile-long blood vessel pipeline.

---

**Cardiovascular Complications in Diabetic Patients:**

- Blindness from clots in the arteries of the eyes
- Kidney failure from kidney artery clogging, requiring dialysis
- Gangrene from clogging of the small arteries of the toes
- Heart attacks from clogging of the coronary arteries
- Strokes from clogging of the brain arteries

---

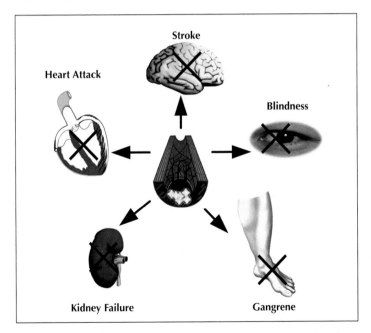

*Cardiovascular complications can occur anywhere in the body of a diabetic.*

153

# How Diabetic Cardiovascular Disease Develops

The key to understanding cardiovascular disease in diabetics is understanding the similarity in the molecular structure of vitamin C and sugar (glucose) molecules. This similarity leads to metabolic confusion with severe consequences:

**Column A** on the opposite page shows that the cells of our blood vessel walls contain tiny biological pumps specialized for pumping sugar and — at the same time — vitamin C molecules from the bloodstream into the blood vessel wall. In a healthy person, these pumps transport an optimum amount of sugar and vitamin C molecules into the blood vessel wall, enabling normal function of the wall and, thus, preventing cardiovascular disease.

**Column B** shows the situation of a diabetic patient. Because of the high sugar concentration in the blood, the sugar and vitamin C pumps are overloaded with sugar molecules. This leads to an overload of sugar and, at the same time, to a deficiency of vitamin C inside the blood vessel walls. The consequence of these mechanisms is a thickening of the walls throughout the blood vessel pipeline, which puts organs at risk for infarctions.

**Column C** shows the decisive measure for preventing cardiovascular complications in diabetes. The optimum daily intake of selected cellular nutrients — in particular vitamin C — helps to restore the balance between vitamin C and sugar metabolism inside the cells of the pancreas, blood vessel walls and other organs.

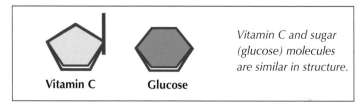

**Vitamin C**     **Glucose**

*Vitamin C and sugar (glucose) molecules are similar in structure.*

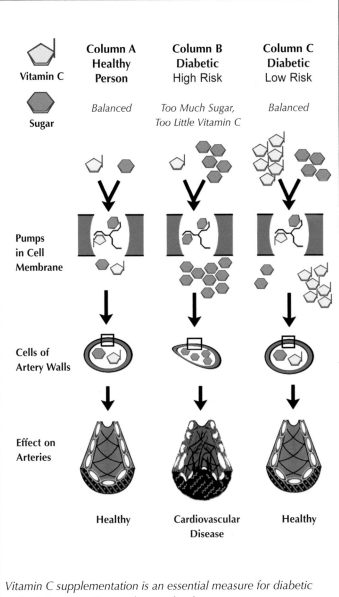

*Vitamin C supplementation is an essential measure for diabetic patients in preventing cardiovascular disease.*

# A Clinical Study Documents Vitamin C Lowers Blood Sugar and Insulin Requirements

Clinical studies show that in diabetic patients, vitamin C contributes not only to the prevention of cardiovascular complications, but also helps to normalize the imbalance in glucose metabolism. Professor R. Pfleger and his colleagues from the University of Vienna published the results of a remarkable clinical study. It showed that diabetic patients taking 300-500 mg of vitamin C a day could significantly improve glucose balance. Blood sugar levels could be lowered on average by 30%, daily insulin requirements by 27% and sugar excretion in the urine could be almost eliminated.

It is amazing that this study was published in 1937 in a leading European journal of internal medicine. If the results of this important study had been followed up and documented in medical textbooks, millions of lives could have been saved and cardiovascular disease would no longer threaten diabetic patients.

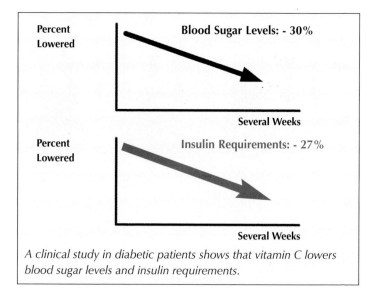

*A clinical study in diabetic patients shows that vitamin C lowers blood sugar levels and insulin requirements.*

# A Clinical Study Documents More Vitamin C Means Less Insulin

Diabetic patients can significantly lower their daily insulin requirements by increasing their daily intake of vitamin C. This is the result of a clinical case study conducted at the renowned Stanford University in California. Dr. J.F. Dice, the lead author of the study, was the diabetic patient in this case report. At the beginning of the study, Dr. Dice injected 32 units of insulin per day.

During the three-week study, Dr. Dice gradually increased his daily intake of vitamin C until he reached 11 grams per day by day 23. The vitamin C was divided in small amounts and taken throughout the day to increase its absorption in his body. By day 23, Dr. Dice's insulin requirement had dropped from 32 units to five units per day. Thus, for every additional gram of dietary vitamin C supplementation, he could spare 2.5 insulin units.

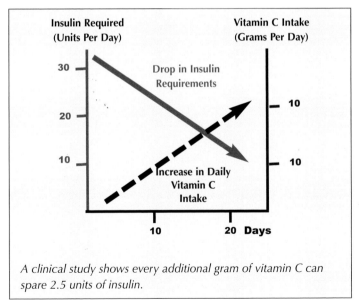

*A clinical study shows every additional gram of vitamin C can spare 2.5 units of insulin.*

# How Diabetic Patients Can Benefit From Dr. Rath's Cellular Health Recommendations

The following section presents a selection of letters from patients with diabetic disorders. I encourage you to share these letters and the contents of this book with anyone you know suffering from diabetes. By doing so, you can help prevent heart attacks, strokes, blindness and other organ failure in those patients.

*Dear Dr. Rath:*

*I started following your cardiovascular vitamin program three months ago.* **I'm 29 years old and was recently diagnosed with Type II Diabetes. Since following your program on a regular basis, I have found my blood glucose level remains around 100 even when under stress, which previously raised my blood glucose level.**

*Your vitamin program and 1-2 extra grams of vitamin C have relieved the primary negative symptoms that I have experienced, such as weakness from low blood sugar levels, pain in the right side from high blood sugar and painful urination from the higher blood sugar levels.*

*I have found only positive results from your program.*

*Sincerely,*
*A.M.*

*Dear Dr. Rath:*

**I would like to share my story with you in the hope that the information will help other diabetics with similar conditions.**
*More importantly, I am hopeful this information will keep other diabetics from ever having to experience the frustration and debilitating pain involved with peripheral neuropathy, as I have.*

**For many years I have been suffering from diabetes and diabetic neuropathy. My toes were turning dark blue and purple, and I did not have any feeling in them. The prognosis was very grim; if my condition did not get better I could lose my toes, if not my feet.**

*I was looking for a treatment that would help this condition. Then I learned about your Cellular Health recommendations. After about a week of following your program, to my delight, my toes became a bright maroon color instead of blue and purple, and much to my amazement, hair was beginning to grow again on my legs, telling me that blood was reaching the hair follicles.*

*By the second week, my legs were not cramping as often or as badly, but by the end of the third week, my feet and ankles were giving me excruciating pain. I mentioned what was happening to me to a friend who is a druggist.* **He happily told me that he believed the nerves were regenerating. Feeling, which has been absent for several years, is coming back in my feet. I can feel the inside of my shoes again. I am now starting the third month on your program.**

**Your Cellular Health recommendations, coupled with my stationery bicycle and insulin adjustments and suggestions from my dietitian, are all elements in helping me fight the battle and win.**

*Very sincerely yours,*
*M.J.*

*Dear Dr. Rath:*

*I am a 55-year-old Caucasian male weighing 154 pounds. I lead a very sedentary life spending most of my time sitting behind a desk in front of a computer.* ***About 20 years ago, I was diagnosed as a Type II (adult onset) diabetic and placed on oral medication and dietary restrictions to control my blood sugar levels.*** *These precautions seemed to work up to about a year ago when my blood sugar went to about 260 and remains fairly steady. This fact caused my physician (an endocrinologist) to change my medication and drastically increase my dosage. He is currently seeing me on a monthly basis in an attempt to stabilize my condition.*

*In February of 1986, I underwent quintuple bypass surgery to remedy severe angina and all the other symptoms of cardiovascular disease. Since the operation, I have not experienced any symptoms such as pain, shortness of breath or irregular heartbeat.* ***I have followed your cardiovascular nutrient program every day as prescribed in your instructions for exactly 2 months, and since approximately 2 weeks ago, I have noticed a dramatic increase in my energy level. I can accomplish much more in my daily work, I find myself eager to stay up late and recently, I found myself out dancing late at night with my wife just as I used to do about 20 years ago.*** *Since nothing in my daily routine has changed except the advent of your program, I must conclude that this newly found "fountain of youth" is a direct result of your program.*

*In closing, I am grateful to your vitamin program for the improvements shown thus far. Please feel free to use this letter, or any part thereof, as a testimonial to your efforts.*

*Sincerely,*
*N.M.*

*Dear Dr. Rath:*

*I am a 69-year-old woman employed full-time in a position that requires close attention to detail and considerable adjustment to time constraints.*

*At the beginning of last year, during my annual physical examination, my physician stated that **I had developed glucose intolerance and that the ultimate result would be diabetes unless I immediately began countermeasures.***

*I then met with a diabetic counselor, and gave her all the information that I possessed concerning your cardiovascular micronutrient program. Following this consultation, I started your program. I also modified my diet, began to exercise regularly and have lost a substantial amount of weight.*

***Now, one year later, my doctor informs me that my diabetic condition is in full remission. Furthermore, my blood pressure is in the normal range, my blood tests are all excellent, my energy has noticeably increased and my general condition is once again first rate.***

*Dr. Rath, I attribute the turnaround in my health to your vitamin program.*

*Thank you.*
*M.B.*

# Clinical Studies Documenting the Benefits of Dr. Rath's Cellular Health Recommendations in Diabetes

Dr. Rath's Cellular Health recommendations were tested in a clinical pilot study with 10 patients suffering from adult onset diabetes (Diabetes Type II). Before the study, after two months, after four months and after six months, blood tests were conducted to measure the effect of my nutrient program on blood sugar levels (glucose), as well as on the long-term diabetes indicator Hb-A1 (sugar-coated hemoglobin).

After six months following my Cellular Health recommendations developed for diabetic patients, the blood sugar levels had dropped from an average of 155 mg/dl at the beginning of the study to an average of 120 at the end of the study. This meant a drop of 23% in blood sugar levels — achieved by a natural approach that provides essential nutrients to correct imbalances in millions of body cells.

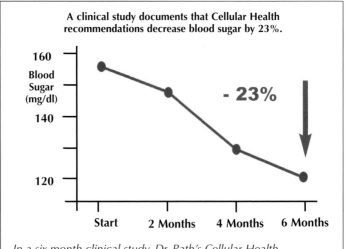

*In a six-month clinical study, Dr. Rath's Cellular Health recommendations lowered the blood sugar levels of diabetic patients by an average of 23%.*

The long-term indicator for diabetes in the blood of diabetic patients was also lowered. After the diabetic patients followed my nutrient program for half a year, their Hb-A1 blood values dropped by an average of 9.3%.

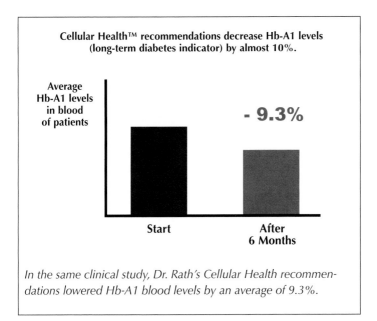

**Cellular Health™ recommendations decrease Hb-A1 levels (long-term diabetes indicator) by almost 10%.**

Average Hb-A1 levels in blood of patients

**- 9.3%**

Start

After 6 Months

*In the same clinical study, Dr. Rath's Cellular Health recommendations lowered Hb-A1 blood levels by an average of 9.3%.*

Further independent studies in which components of my Cellular Health recommendations were tested are summarized below:

| Cellular Nutrients Tested | Reference |
| --- | --- |
| Vitamin C | Mann, Som, Stankova, Stepp and Hirashima |
| Vitamin E | Paolisso |
| Magnesium | McNair and Mather |
| Chromium | Liu and Riales |

# Cellular Health Recommendations for Patients With Diabetes

In addition to the Basic Cellular Health recommendations described in Chapter One, I recommend that patients with diabetes and diabetic complications take the following cellular bioenergy factors in higher dosages:

- **Vitamin C:** corrects cellular imbalances caused by elevated blood sugar levels, contributes to lower insulin requirements, decreases glucose elimination in the urine and, above all, protects the artery walls

- **Vitamin E:** provides antioxidant protection and protection of the cell membranes

- **Vitamins B1, B2, B3, B5, B6, B12 and Biotin:** bio-energy carriers of cellular metabolism, improved metabolic efficacy, particularly of the liver cells, and the central unit of the body metabolism

- **Chromium:** a trace element that functions as a biocatalyst for optimum metabolism of glucose and insulin

- **Inositol and Choline:** components of lecithin, which are important components of each cell membrane and essential for optimum metabolic transport and supply of each cell with nutrients and other biomolecules

**Please note:** The most important goal is to provide optimum protection for your artery walls, not to completely replace your insulin. In many cases, particularly in patients with *inherited* (juvenile) insulin deficiency, this will not be possible.

# Notes

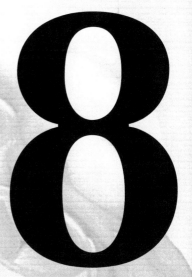

# 8

# Specific Cardiovascular Problems

Dr. Rath's Cellular Health Recommendations for Prevention and Adjunct Therapy

- The Facts about Angina Pectoris

- Dr. Rath's Cellular Health Recommendations Help:
  - Ameliorate Angina Pectoris
  - Patients After a Heart Attack
  - Patients Undergoing Coronary Bypass Surgery
  - Patients Undergoing Coronary Angioplasty

# The Facts About Angina Pectoris

Angina pectoris is the typical alarm signal for atherosclerotic deposits in the coronary arteries and decreased blood supply to millions of heart muscle cells. Angina pectoris typically manifests as a sharp pain in the middle of the chest, which frequently radiates into the left arm. Because there are many atypical forms of angina pectoris, I advise you to consult with a physician about any form of unclear chest pain.

My Cellular Health recommendations can help to improve the blood supply to the heart muscle cells by providing oxygen and nutrients, thereby decreasing angina pectoris. Several essential nutrients in this program work together to achieve this aim. The most important mechanisms for increasing blood supply to heart muscle tissue are the following:

- **Widening of arteries:** An optimum supply of vitamin C and magnesium, as well as the natural amino acid arginine, aid in widening the coronary arteries and increase blood supply through the coronary arteries to the heart muscle cells.

- **Improved blood pumping:** Carnitine, coenzyme Q-10, B vitamins, certain minerals and trace elements improve the performance of the heart muscle cells, the pumping function of the heart, the pressure by which the blood is pumped through the coronary arteries and, thereby, the supply of oxygen and nutrients to the heart muscle cells.

- **Reversal of coronary deposits:** Over a period of many months, vitamin C, lysine and proline initiate the healing process of the artery walls and the decrease of atherosclerotic deposits by the mechanisms described in detail earlier in this book.

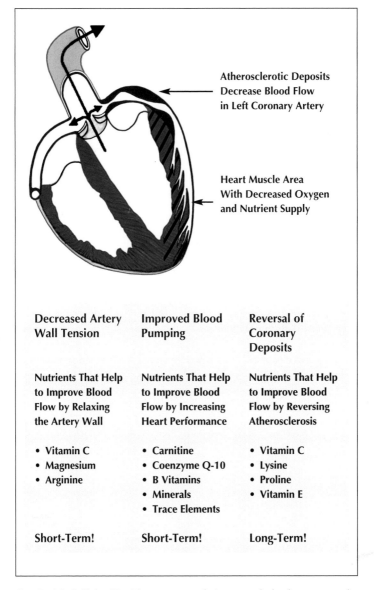

**Atherosclerotic Deposits Decrease Blood Flow in Left Coronary Artery**

**Heart Muscle Area With Decreased Oxygen and Nutrient Supply**

| Decreased Artery Wall Tension | Improved Blood Pumping | Reversal of Coronary Deposits |
|---|---|---|
| Nutrients That Help to Improve Blood Flow by Relaxing the Artery Wall | Nutrients That Help to Improve Blood Flow by Increasing Heart Performance | Nutrients That Help to Improve Blood Flow by Reversing Atherosclerosis |
| • Vitamin C<br>• Magnesium<br>• Arginine | • Carnitine<br>• Coenzyme Q-10<br>• B Vitamins<br>• Minerals<br>• Trace Elements | • Vitamin C<br>• Lysine<br>• Proline<br>• Vitamin E |
| Short-Term! | Short-Term! | Long-Term! |

*Dr. Rath's Cellular Health recommendations can help decrease and prevent angina pectoris.*

169

# How Dr. Rath's Cellular Health Recommendations Can Help Patients With Angina Pectoris

The following section presents a selection of letters from patients with coronary heart disease and angina pectoris. This book documents the success of my Cellular Health recommendations, which enable angina pectoris patients around the world to take advantage of this medical breakthrough and improve their quality of life.

---

*Dear Dr. Rath:*

*I am so happy to tell you about the use of your cardiovascular health program and how I feel that it has saved my life. Last September, I had gone to the university to watch a football game and could not make it up the steps in the stadium despite wearing a nitroglycerin patch, and **by October last year, I could not walk 100 yards without the pain of angina.***

***I found out about your discovery and took it triple strength four times a day for three weeks and by Thanksgiving, I had forgotten I had a heart problem. Now, in July of this year, I am working without pain and feeling super!***

*Too bad you did not have the patent before I had undergone two bypass surgeries.*

*Thanks for more life,*
*J.G.*

---

# How Patients Can Be Helped By Cellular Health Recommendations After a Heart Attack

The following are letters from patients who benefited from my Cellular Health recommendations after suffering a heart attack. Please share this information with anyone you know with a similar health condition. You may help prevent further heart attacks.

---

*Dear Dr. Rath:*

*In January of this year, I began experiencing chest pains when exercising. In April, my doctor told me, on the basis of an EKG, that I had suffered a heart attack. He continued prescribing a beta-blocker, which I had been taking for high blood pressure for many years.*

*In May, I started following your cardiovascular vitamin program and also went on a very strict vegetarian, no-fat diet. My chest pain during exercise began to lessen after just two weeks of this regimen. I have now been on a diet and your vitamin program for 2 months, and I now have no chest pain or breathlessness at all, even when cycling or walking energetically for several hours at a time. I also feel better than I have felt for years, with lots of energy and high spirits.*

*My confidence level in my heart condition is so good that I no longer carry nitroglycerin pills with me when setting out on a bicycle ride or a walk. I feel young and bright. Since the only change in my lifestyle has been your cardiovascular health program and diet, I have to say that one or both of these factors have caused this dramatic change in my health. For what it is worth, I tend to think that the combination of both these factors together is what has caused my health to improve.*

*Yours truly,*
*K.P.*

---

*Dear Dr. Rath:*

**My dad was diagnosed with blockages of the heart in October of last year. He also suffered from angina and arrhythmia.** *He could not walk a block without concern for his ability to make it home again. My dad was concerned for his life because he had two ischemic events (four years ago). Along with being diabetic and 80 years of age, his medical advisors ruled out an invasive procedure as a remedy.*

*When I was first made aware of your breakthrough non-invasive therapy, I could not believe our good fortune. Immediately, we placed Dad on your cardiovascular vitamin program. Within a day, he reported good results. "I feel good!" was his response after the first day. The second day, he told me that his energy level had increased significantly. "I was able to work in the garage all day today without getting tired." **The third day Dad had walked a block and returned without difficulty – no pains, fatigue, or apprehension.***

*The chest pains went away by December. In January, on our way to the cardiologist's office, Dad, having forgotten his essential nutrients for his doctor's inspection and review, ran back into the house to retrieve them. I got so excited by the event that I immediately started calling people on my car phone to share with them what I had just witnessed – a miracle!*

**My dad's heart no longer skips a beat, his angina is gone,** *and his blood flows freely when he proudly donates blood samples. His doctors are amazed with his newfound state of health. And we are very, very happy. Last week my dad took a 10 block walk without difficulty; he is proud and grateful.*

*Thank you, Dr. Rath. Your research has given my dad back his life.*

*Sincerely,*
*M.T.*

# Dr. Rath's Cellular Health Recommendations for Patients Undergoing Coronary Bypass Surgery

## What Is a Coronary Bypass Operation?

A coronary bypass operation becomes necessary if one or more coronary arteries have developed severe atherosclerotic deposits that threaten to clog the arteries and cause a heart attack. In order to avoid a heart attack, a coronary bypass operation is frequently performed. Surgically, a bypass is constructed around the atherosclerotic deposits in order to guarantee unrestricted blood flow to all parts of the heart muscle in those areas beyond the coronary deposits.

During a bypass operation, a vein is generally taken from the leg and re-implanted in the heart as a bypass blood vessel. Normally, one end of the bypass is attached to the aorta and the other end is attached to the coronary artery beyond the location narrowed by atherosclerotic deposits. Other bypass

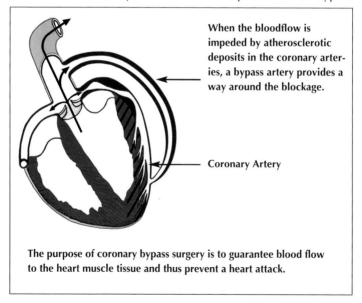

When the bloodflow is impeded by atherosclerotic deposits in the coronary arteries, a bypass artery provides a way around the blockage.

Coronary Artery

**The purpose of coronary bypass surgery is to guarantee blood flow to the heart muscle tissue and thus prevent a heart attack.**

*The reason bypass surgery is performed*

surgery procedures use smaller arteries in the vicinity of the heart to construct a bypass and improve blood supply to the heart muscle.

I am often asked whether a coronary bypass operation can be avoided by following my Cellular Health reccommendations. As documented in this book, the operation can, in many cases, be postponed or cancelled. However, in other cases, the atherosclerotic deposits have grown so much that a bypass operation is unavoidable. In any case, the decision can only be made together with your cardiologist. But even if a bypass operation has become inevitable, you should start immediately following my nutrient program to improve the long-term success of this operation and to prevent further damage.

### What Are Problems After a Coronary Bypass Operation?

The overall success of a coronary artery bypass operation is threatened by two main problems:

- **Blood clots:** Blood clots can form in the bypass blood vessels, cutting off the blood flow. This complication normally occurs immediately after the operation. If untreated, the blood clot will completely cut off blood flow through the bypass blood vessel and make the previous operation ineffective.

- **Atherosclerotic deposits:** The greatest threat to the long-term success of a coronary bypass operation is the development of atherosclerotic deposits in the newly implanted bypass blood vessels. Even though the bypass blood vessel is generally a vein, the same lesions and cracks can develop as in the arteries if they are not protected by an optimum intake of vitamins and other essential nutrients. This triggers atherosclerotic deposits similar to those in the coronary arteries and, after several years, can require a second bypass operation.

On the following pages, I have summarized the recent progress in the field of Cellular Medicine.

**Complication No. 1:**    Blood Clot Formation in Bypass Vessels

Coronary Bypass Blood Vessels

Blood Clot Blocking Blood Flow
in Bypass

**Complication No. 2:**    New Deposits Develop in Bypass
Grafts and Old Deposits in
Coronary Arteries Continue to Grow

Old Deposits

New Deposits

Dr. Rath's Cellular Health Recommendations Can Improve Short-
Term and Long-Term Success Rate After Coronary Bypass Surgery:

Nutrients Decreasing Risk for Blood Clotting:
• Vitamin C      • Beta-carotene
• Vitamin E      • Arginine

Nutrients Decreasing Risk for New Deposits:
• Vitamin C      • Proline
• Lysine         • Antioxidants

*Obstacles to the long-term success of coronary bypass surgery and how
Dr. Rath's Cellular Health recommendations help to prevent them*

> *The average time that passes between the first bypass oper-*
> *ation of a patient and the second bypass surgery is about 10*
> *years. The fact that a second bypass is the rule, and not the*
> *exception, shows that the causes of bypass atherosclerosis*
> *are insufficiently understood by conventional medicine.*

## How Dr. Rath's Cellular Health Recommendations Improve the Long-Term Success of Coronary Bypass Surgery

There are several ways in which nutritional supplements help to maintain healthy bypass blood vessels and improve the quality of life after bypass surgery.

- **Preventing blood clot formation in bypass blood vessels:** Vitamin C, vitamin E and beta-carotene have all been shown to help prevent the formation of blood clots. Vitamin C has also been shown to help dissolve already existing blood clots. Patients on "Coumadin" and other blood thinners should inform their doctors when starting my program so that additional tests for blood coagulation can be done and less blood-thinning medication can be prescribed.

- **Preventing atherosclerotic deposits in bypass blood vessels:** The vitamins and other essential nutrients recommended for the prevention and adjunct reversal of atherosclerotic deposits in coronary arteries are also beneficial for preventing the development of atherosclerotic deposits in bypass blood vessels. The most important among these essential nutrients are vitamin C, vitamin E and the amino acids lysine and proline.

If you are scheduled for a bypass operation, I recommend that you start with these Cellular Health recommendations as soon as possible. In this way, you can make sure that the cells of your heart, blood vessels and other body tissues already hold an optimum level of vitamins and other bioenergy molecules during and immediately after the operation. This is the best natural way to optimize the healing process.

The following is a testimonial from a patient who supplemented with my Cellular Health recommendations after coronary bypass surgery:

---

*Dear Dr. Rath:*

**I read your book about a year ago after I was told I had severe blockage of the coronary arteries, and I had a triple bypass operation. At that time, I started following your cardiovascular vitamin program.**

**All of my check-ups since my surgery have been outstanding. I attribute much of the good news to your program.**

*For a long time, I have maintained an opinion that there was a better answer to heart disease than the standard American Medical Association medical approach. Thank you for finding the answer and making it available to all of us who need it.*

*Sincerely,*
*C.S.*

---

You will find many more letters from coronary heart disease patients in the chapters on cardiovascular disease, angina pectoris and heart attacks.

# Dr. Rath's Cellular Health Recommendations for Patients Undergoing Coronary Angioplasty

## What Is a Coronary Angioplasty?

In contrast to coronary bypass surgery, coronary angioplasty is the "rotor-rooter" approach to removing atherosclerotic deposits mechanically. This approach generally involves an inflatable balloon or, more recently, laser or scraping methods. Generally, a catheter is inserted into the leg artery and moved forward through the aorta until the catheter tip reaches the coronary artery close to the deposits. At this point, a balloon at the tip of the catheter is inflated with high pressure and squeezes the atherosclerotic deposits flat against the wall of the arteries. In many cases, the blood flow through the coronary artery can be improved by this procedure.

All angioplasty procedures damage the inside of the coronary arteries, sometimes over a distance of several inches. It is, therefore, not surprising that the rate of complications of this procedure is sobering. In more than 30% of cases a restenosis occurs, leading to the clogging of the coronary artery within a time as short as six months.

The most serious complication during the procedure is the rupturing of the wall of the coronary artery, requiring immediate bypass surgery. Following the procedure, blood clots and small pieces of artery wall tissue can lead to a clogging of the coronary artery. Long-term complications include the overgrowth of scar tissue inside the coronary artery and the continued development of atherosclerotic deposits.

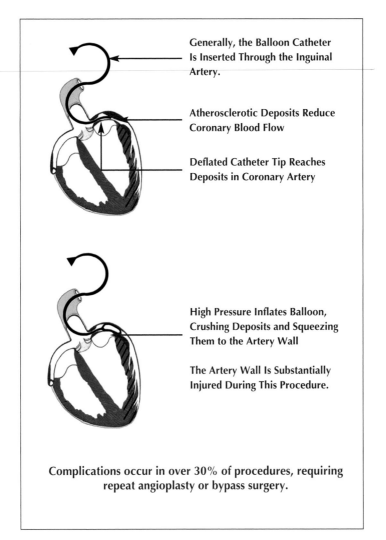

Generally, the Balloon Catheter Is Inserted Through the Inguinal Artery.

Atherosclerotic Deposits Reduce Coronary Blood Flow

Deflated Catheter Tip Reaches Deposits in Coronary Artery

High Pressure Inflates Balloon, Crushing Deposits and Squeezing Them to the Artery Wall

The Artery Wall Is Substantially Injured During This Procedure.

Complications occur in over 30% of procedures, requiring repeat angioplasty or bypass surgery.

*Angioplasty inevitably causes substantial damage to the artery wall.*

## How Dr. Rath's Cellular Health Recommendations Can Help to Improve the Success Rate of Angioplasty

My Cellular Health recommendations can help patients scheduled for coronary angioplasty in different ways. In some cases, they can help decrease angina pectoris and other signs of coronary heart disease to an extent that your doctor will suggest postponement of the angioplasty procedure. In other cases, your doctor will advise you to have the procedure to minimize your risk of a heart attack. In any case, you should follow the advice of your doctor. At the same time, I recommend that you start these Cellular Health recommendations as soon as possible and inform your doctor about it. If you have already undergone coronary angioplasty, my recommendations can help you to improve the long-term success of this procedure.

- **Vitamin C** accelerates healing of the wounds in the coronary arteries caused by the angioplasty procedure.

- **Lysine and proline** also help restore the artery wall structure and, at the same time, decrease the risk of fatty deposit formation.

- **Vitamin E and vitamin C** help control the overshooting formation of scar tissue from the uncontrolled growth of arterial wall muscle cells.

- **Vitamin C, vitamin E and beta-carotene** decrease the risk of blood clot formation and provide important antioxidant protection.

## Further Health Information Related to Dr. Rath's Cellular Health Recommendations and Angioplasty

Research and clinical studies have confirmed the important role of different components of my Cellular Health recommendations in decreasing the risk of the clogging of coronary arteries after angioplasty:

Dr. Samuel DeMaio, while at Emory University in Atlanta, Georgia, studied patients with coronary heart disease who had undergone coronary angioplasty. After this procedure, one group of patients received 1,200 International Units of vitamin E as a nutritional supplement. The control group received no additional vitamin E. After four months, the patients who had received vitamin E showed a 15% decrease in the rate of coronary restenosis, compared to those patients without vitamin E supplementation.

My colleague Dr. Aleksandra Niedzwiecki and her collaborators showed that vitamin C decreases the overgrowth of the smooth muscle cells of the artery wall and helps to control one of the most frequent factors responsible for the failure of angioplasty procedures. Animal experiments conducted with vitamin C and vitamin E by Dr. Gilberto Nunes and his colleagues confirmed these observations.

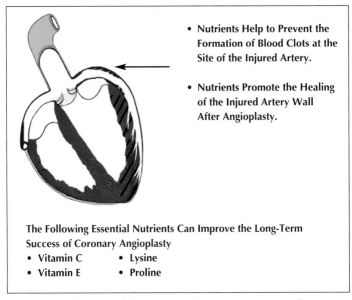

- **Nutrients Help to Prevent the Formation of Blood Clots at the Site of the Injured Artery.**

- **Nutrients Promote the Healing of the Injured Artery Wall After Angioplasty.**

**The Following Essential Nutrients Can Improve the Long-Term Success of Coronary Angioplasty**
- **Vitamin C**
- **Vitamin E**
- **Lysine**
- **Proline**

*Dr. Rath's Cellular Health recommendations can improve the success rate of coronary angioplasty.*

185

My Cellular Health recommendations include a selection of essential nutrients that work synergistically in helping to improve the long-term success of coronary angioplasty. Of course, you can increase the amounts of specific vitamins, such as vitamin C and vitamin E, to further enhance this effect.

The following is a letter from a patient who supplemented with these Cellular Health recommendations after having coronary angioplasty. More letters from coronary heart disease patients are documented in previous chapters.

---

*Dear Dr. Rath:*

**Your vitamin program has done so much to improve the quality of my life healthwise that I would like to share it with others.** *I was 83 years old last February. I was having so much angina pain that my family doctor sent me to a cardiologist, who did an angio- plasty. In the meantime, my 78-year-old husband had a triple by- pass followed by a stroke. I had to get better to take care of him, but I continued to have the same pains.* **A second cardiologist did angioplasty in August last year, which did not help, so in September I had a double bypass and needed a third.**

*My son started me on your cellular nutrient program. In January of this year, I was still having angina due to an artery they were unable to bypass.* **After 3 months, I quit having pains due to stress or strain or excitement and now, after six months, I feel great and do almost as much physically as I did 5 or 10 years ago.**

*My husband, although hampered by his stroke, also enjoys better health with your cardiovascular health program.*

*Sincerely,*
*L.W.*

---

# Clinical Studies With Cellular Nutrients in Angina Pectoris Patients

Additional reports from patients with angina pectoris about health improvements with selected components of Dr. Rath's Cellular Health recommendations are documented in Chapter Two of this book.

The following table lists additional clinical studies document-ing the health benefits of cellular nutrients in patients with coronary heart disease and angina pectoris:

| Cellular Nutrients Tested | References |
|---|---|
| Vitamin C and Vitamin E | Riemersma |
| Beta-carotene | Riemersma |
| Carnitine | Ferrari and Opie |
| Coenzyme Q-10 | Folkers and Kamikawa |
| Magnesium | Iseri and Teo |

*Dear Dr. Rath:*

*I started following your cardiovascular nutrient program last August after I was diagnosed as having severe heart disease. **I had angina for 8 years. Now, nearly a year later, I feel fine and have very slight angina infrequently, plus I walk 3.6 miles daily and don't have any restrictions.***

*Sincerely,*
*M.B.*

---

*Dear Dr. Rath:*

***Since following your vitamin program, I have noticed a significant increase in my physical and mental health. I have no present indications of angina, and my ability to walk vigorously around the hills that are in my neighborhood is most encouraging. No huffing and puffing and pausing to catch my breath, as before.***

*I am able to walk around my neighborhood hills without interrupting the rhythm and flow of my conversation. I also pursue a very modest weight loss program, eating much less than before — with no loss of energy.*

*I feel that your program is most significant in all of this.*

*Sincerely yours,*
*R.A.*

---

*Dear Dr. Rath:*

*I had been having chest pain (angina pectoris) for several years on the average of about every three weeks. **Since I started your vitamin program over 90 days ago, I have only had chest pain one time, which was about three weeks after starting your program.***

*I feel that proper nutrition can prevent 80% of our health problems.*

*Sincerely,*
*B.T.*

188

# Notes

# 9

# External and Inherited Cardiovascular Risks

**Dr. Rath's Cellular Health Recommendations for Prevention and Adjunct Therapy**

- Unhealthy Diet
- Smoking
- Stress
- Hormonal Contraceptives
- Pharmaceutical Drugs
- Dialysis
- Surgery
- Inherited Risk Factors for Cardiovascular Disease

# Unhealthy Diet

The basis of any natural cardiovascular health program is a healthy diet. For many generations, the diets of our ancestors shaped the metabolism of our bodies today. By understanding our ancestors' diets, we have learned what is best for our bodies now. Their diets were rich in cereal, fruits, vegetables and other plant nutrition high in fiber and vitamins. They ate considerably less fat and sugar than we do today. Conversely, the average diet in industrialized countries imposes a heavy metabolic burden on our bodies. Certain inherited disorders put our bodies at further risk.

My Cellular Health recommendations have been shown to optimize metabolism. This is particularly important for fat metabolism in our bodies. My nutrient program can help you to:

- **Lower cholesterol production in your body**
- **Optimize the metabolism of fat molecules in your cells**
- **Optimize the elimination of fat from your body**
- **Protect fat molecules from oxidation**

It is important to understand that certain vitamins are literally used up in the degradation process of these fat molecules. For every molecule of cholesterol, whether it is produced in the body or comes from the diet, our bodies use up one molecule of vitamin C in an enzymatic reaction in the liver.

In this way, high cholesterol and triglyceride levels can contribute to chronic vitamin depletion in the body. Thus, it is important to understand that an increased cardiovascular risk is not primarily the result of too many fat molecules in the diet, but is primarily due to the systematic depletion of the vitamin reserves in our bodies from an overburdened fat metabolism. As a consequence of chronic vitamin depletion, the artery walls are weakened and cardiovascular disease develops.

Besides too much fat, there are other dangers in our diets. Residues from herbicides, pesticides and chemical preservatives are present in essentially every meal we eat. These toxic substances have to be detoxified in the liver. Vitamin C and other components of my Cellular Health recommendations are essential cofactors for the detoxification of these substances in our bodies.

**My recommendations:**

Eat a prudent diet. Watch your body weight and exercise regularly. A healthy diet is rich in plant nutrition and contains abundant vitamins and fiber substances. Try to avoid consuming too much fat and sweetened food. Above all, avoid chronic depletion of your body's vitamin reserves by following my Cellular Health recommendations on a daily basis.

# Smoking

While it is known that smoking dramatically increases the risk for cardiovascular disease, the underlying reason is often unclear. Cigarette smoke contains millions of free radicals, which are aggressive molecules that damage the cells of our blood vessels and other organs and accelerate biological rusting. Free radicals and other toxic substances in cigarette smoke reach the bloodstream via the lungs. These noxious substances can damage the blood vessel pipeline along its entire length of 60,000 miles.
In the body's defense against these aggressive molecules, antioxidants are used up. Among all antioxidants, vitamin C is the first one to be destroyed. With the body's vitamin reserves depleted, cardiovascular disease starts in the blood vessel system — just as in early scurvy.

Now we understand why atherosclerosis in smokers is not limited to the coronary arteries and why damage occurs in the arteries and capillaries throughout the body. "Smoker's foot" is typical, requiring toes or a foot to be amputated.

My Cellular Health recommendations include numerous antioxidants, which are able to neutralize free radicals contained in cigarette smoke and help prevent damage to the artery wall and other body tissues.

**My recommendations:**

If you still smoke, it is worth the effort to stop. Perhaps this chapter will help you become aware of how much damage you actually cause in your body by smoking. For smokers and ex-smokers, my recommendation is the same: optimize your daily intake of natural antioxidants, preferably in the form of my Cellular Health recommendations.

# Stress

Chronic physical and psychological stress increases the risk for cardiovascular disease. What is the underlying biochemical mechanism for this phenomenon?

During physical or emotional stress, the body produces high amounts of the stress hormone adrenaline. For every molecule of adrenaline produced, the body needs one molecule of vitamin C as the catalyst, and these molecules are destroyed in this process. Thus, long-term physical or emotional stress can lead to a severe depletion of the body's reservoir of vitamin C. If vitamin C is not supplemented in the diet, the cardiovascular system is weakened and atherosclerosis develops.

These facts also explain why spouses frequently die soon one after another. The loss of a partner results in long-term emotional stress and fast vitamin depletion in the body, thereby increasing the risk for a heart attack. We have to understand that it is not the emotional stress itself that causes the heart attack, rather, it is the biochemical consequence of the depletion of the vitamin reserves in the body.

**My recommendations:**

Try to find time to relax. Schedule time to unwind just as you schedule your professional appointments. In the case of severe emotional problems, you may also benefit from professional consultation. Irrespective of these steps, make sure that you supplement your body's reservoir with vitamins and other components of my Cellular Health recommendations.

# Hormonal Contraceptives and Estrogen Replacement Therapy

Long-term intake of estrogen and other hormones — both as hormonal contraception and hormone replacement therapy during menopause — cause a depletion of vitamins and other cellular nutrients in the body. This is the reason why women taking these hormones have an increased risk for heart attacks, strokes and other forms of cardiovascular disease.

Several studies show that women taking hormonal contraceptives ("the Pill") significantly increase their risk for cardiovascular disease. In 1972, Dr. Briggs reported in the scientific journal *Nature* that women taking hormonal contraceptives had significantly lower vitamin C blood levels than normal. In another study, Dr. Rivers confirmed these results and concluded that vitamin C depletion was associated with the estrogen hormone. The fact is that long-term use of hormonal contraceptives decreases the body pool of vitamin C and other essential nutrients, such as B vitamins and calcium. Thus, it is not the birth control pill itself that increases the risk for cardiovascular disease, but the associated depletion of the vitamin body pool, which weakens the blood vessel wall.

It came as no surprise that the largest clinical study designed to show the possible benefits of hormone replacement therapy conducted in more than 16,000 women had to be prematurely stopped because of the significantly increased risk for heart attacks, thrombosis and other complications.

**My recommendations:**

If you have been taking hormonal birth control pills or have undergone hormone repacement therapy, make sure that you start following my Cellular Health recommendations to re-supplement your body's vitamin pool and prevent its future depletion.

# Pharmaceutical Drugs

Almost all the prescription drugs currently taken by millions of people lead to a gradual depletion of vitamins and other essential cellular nutrients in the body. Drugs are generally synthetic, non-natural substances that we absorb in our bodies. Our bodies recognize these synthetic drugs as "toxic," just like any other non-natural substance.

Thus, all synthetic drugs have to be "detoxified" by the liver in order to eliminate them from our bodies. This detoxification process requires vitamin C and other cellular nutrients as cofactors. Many of these essential nutrients are used up in biological (enzymatic) reactions during this detoxification process. One of the most common ways for eliminating drugs from our bodies is called "hydroxylation." The strongest "hydroxylating agent" in our bodies is vitamin C, which is literally destroyed during this detoxification process.

Thus, long-term use of many synthetic prescription drugs leads to a chronic vitamin depletion in the body, a form of early scurvy and the onset of cardiovascular disease.

Another way in which certain prescription drugs, such as the cholesterol-lowering agent "Cholestyramine," contribute to vitamin depletion is their binding to vitamins in the intestine. This prevents optimum absorption of vitamins from the digestive tract into the bloodstream and body.

Prescription drugs can also deplete the body's reservoir of certain essential nutrients by interfering with the natural production of these essential nutrients in the body. "Lovastatin," "Pravastatin" and other cholesterol-lowering drugs in the statin category inhibit the production of cholesterol in the cells of the body. Unfortunately, they also decrease the production rate of important natural molecules, such as coenzyme Q-10 (ubiquinone).

Karl Folkers, MD, of the University of Texas at Austin, reported that heart failure patients with low baseline coenzyme Q-10 levels could experience life-threatening cardiovascular complications when taking these cholesterol-lowering drugs because of a decrease of coenzyme Q-10 in the body.

## Diuretic Drugs

Taking diuretic drugs can significantly increase your risk for cardiovascular disease. Diuretics flush not only water from the body, but also water-soluble vitamins and other essential nutrients. I described this mechanism in detail in Chapter Five. The importance of regular supplementation of these vitamins and other essential nutrients in patients taking diuretics cannot be overemphasized.

## My recommendations:

If you are taking any prescription drugs, I recommend that you begin immediately with my Cellular Health recommendations. If you are on diuretic medication, the daily supplementation of water-soluble vitamins, minerals and other essential nutrients is imperative. Follow the recommendations in this book, and inform your doctor about it.

# Dialysis

Several investigations have shown that patients undergoing long-term dialysis have an increased risk of cardiovascular disease. This is not surprising, since dialysis eliminates not only the body's waste products from the blood, but also many vitamins and other essential nutrients. If these essential nutrients are not resupplemented, chronic dialysis will lead to a gradual depletion of water-soluble vitamins and other essential nutrients throughout the body, thereby triggering atherosclerosis, heart failure, irregular heartbeat or other forms of cardiovascular disease.

**My recommendations:**

If you are undergoing dialysis, you should immediately start following my Cellular Health recommendations. If you know a dialysis patient, please make sure that you share the information in this book with them; you could help prolong a life.

# Surgery

Patients undergoing an operation should make sure that the cells of their bodies are optimally supplied with vitamins and other cellular nutrients. Each operation results in extraordinary physical and psychological stress for the patient. Preparation for the operation, the operation itself and the healing process result in high stress for several weeks, and can lead to serious vitamin depletion in your body at its time of greatest need.

Moreover, each operation is associated with damage to body tissue. The speed at which the operation wound heals is directly related to the rate at which collagen and other connective tissue molecules are formed to heal it. Vitamin C and other components of my Cellular Health recommendations are your best natural option for optimizing the production of collagen molecules and speeding up the healing phase after an operation.

This nutrient program also helps to protect against oxidative damage during operations. A variety of surgical procedures require external (extra-corporal) circulation. During a bypass operation, the heartbeat is stopped and blood circulation is maintained by a heart-lung machine. During this external circulation, the patient's blood is artificially enriched with oxygen. High concentrations of oxygen can lead to tissue damage in the artery walls and other body tissues (reperfusion injury).

My Cellular Health recommendations are rich in antioxidants and can minimize the risks of oxidative damage during an operation. Taken before, during and after hospitalization, these cellular nutrients help to prevent nutrient depletion and the damage associated with it. For this reason, leading medical schools are now routinely recommending vitamin supplementation to their surgery patients.

The following table summarizes some of the studies with specific components of my Cellular Health recommendations in decreasing different risk factors for cardiovascular disease:

| Depletion of Cellular Nutrients | Reference |
|---|---|
| Blood Fats | Ginter, Harwood and Sokoloff |
| Smoking | Chow, Halliwell, Lehr and Riemersma |
| Stress | Levine |
| "The Pill" | Briggs and Rivers |
| Dialysis | Blumberg |
| Prescription Drugs | Halliwell and Clemetson |

# Inherited Risk Factors for Cardiovascular Disease

I am frequently asked whether these Cellular Health recommendations can also help decrease the risk of inherited risk factors. In many cases, the answer is "yes." Besides the external risk factors discussed in the previous section, the inherited, or genetic, risks constitute the other large group of cardiovascular risk factors.

Everyone has heard the statement, "Heart disease runs in our family." Members of these families frequently die in the fourth or fifth decade of their lives. The causes of these early deaths are, at least in part, caused by abnormal genes (molecules of inheritance), which are passed on from generation to generation in that family. Earlier in this book, I described two of the most frequent genetic risk factors — inherited disorders of fat metabolism (high cholesterol, or hypercholesterolemia) and inherited disorders of sugar metabolism (diabetes).

What is important to understand is that this genetic risk is not a death sentence for anyone. The genetic deficiency generally results in an impaired metabolic function at one location or another in our cellular software program. In most cases, this genetic impairment can be compensated for by an increased intake of essential nutrients. As we already know, vitamins and other essential nutrients are cellular biological catalysts, and they are able to speed up impaired biochemical reactions.

It is, then, no surprise that vitamins and other essential nutrients have already been shown to have profound health benefits in patients with genetic disorders.

The following table provides a list of inherited disorders. Patients with these disorders can benefit from following my Cellular Health recommendations.

If you know anyone with one of the following inherited diseases, please introduce the information in this book to them. As you will see from the histories of Alzheimer's and lupus erythematosus patients on the following pages, these patients greatly benefited from following my Cellular Health recommendations. This is even more important considering the fact that conventional medicine has no answers to these serious health problems.

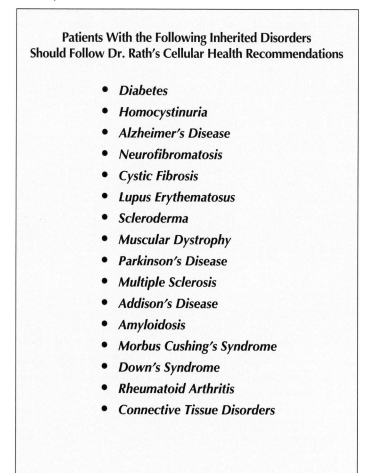

**Patients With the Following Inherited Disorders
Should Follow Dr. Rath's Cellular Health Recommendations**

- *Diabetes*
- *Homocystinuria*
- *Alzheimer's Disease*
- *Neurofibromatosis*
- *Cystic Fibrosis*
- *Lupus Erythematosus*
- *Scleroderma*
- *Muscular Dystrophy*
- *Parkinson's Disease*
- *Multiple Sclerosis*
- *Addison's Disease*
- *Amyloidosis*
- *Morbus Cushing's Syndrome*
- *Down's Syndrome*
- *Rheumatoid Arthritis*
- *Connective Tissue Disorders*

# How Dr. Rath's Cellular Health Recommendations Can Help Decrease Inherited Cardiovascular Risks

Let's take diabetes, for example. With this disease, a genetic defect results in too little production or cellular availability of the insulin hormone. The clinical consequences are discussed in detail in Chapter Seven. Although my Cellular Health recommendations cannot repair defective genes, they can help prevent, or at least delay, the development of diabetic cardiovascular complications.

In the adjacent figure, the defective gene is symbolized as a time bomb. My Cellular Health recommendations cannot make this time bomb disappear. However, they can contribute to defusing it and preventing an "explosion" in the form of a disease appearing.

As documented in this book, for diabetes, cholesterol disorders, Alzheimer's disease, lupus erythematosus and other conditions, my Cellular Health recommendations are an effective therapeutic approach for reducing risks from inherited disorders, and particularly, the development of cardiovascular complications.

The picture on the opposite page summarizes the main factors contributing to your personal cardiovascular risk. Inherited risk factors plus external risk factors determine your overall risk for cardiovascular disease by gradually depleting your body's reservoir of essential nutrients. Most internal and external risk factors are effectively neutralized by an optimum intake of vitamins and other essential nutrients.

You can reduce your cardiovascular risk with two measures:
- Minimizing your external risk factors, such as smoking and diet
- Increasing your daily intake of vitamins and other cellular nutrients

202

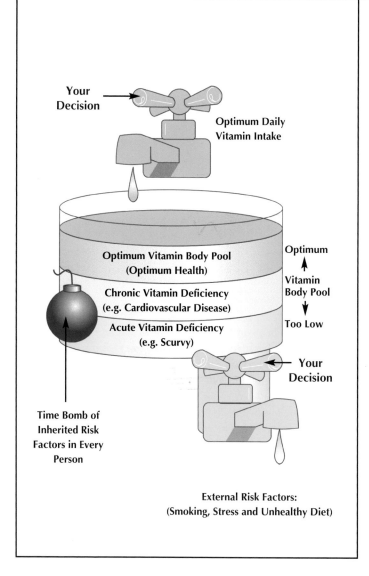

*Maintaining an optimum body pool of cellular nutrients is the key to minimizing inherited cardiovascular risks and enjoying optimum health.*

# How Dr. Rath's Cellular Health Recommendations Can Help Patients With Alzheimer's Disease

Alzheimer's disease is a degenerative condition that leads to the gradual impairment of brain function. Conventional medicine has no therapy for this serious health problem.

*Dear Dr. Rath:*

***My father, who is 84, has Alzheimer's disease.*** *About two months ago, his caregivers attended an Alzheimer's seminar at a nursing home. The seminar reported that some patients had been put on vitamin supplements, which had resulted in improved memory for several patients. We compared ingredients and decided that your cardiovascular vitamin program offered more than what was used at the nursing home.*

***My father has been on this program for two months, and we cannot believe the improvement. His short-term memory is improving, and we can carry on conversations with him again. He is even showing some problem-solving capabilities again.***

*I know these improvements are not measurable from a "pure scientific perspective," but to us it's a blessing to see improvement rather than just deterioration from this terrible disease.*

*On behalf of my father and our family, thank you for your cardiovascular health program.*

*Yours truly,*
*D.C.*

# How Dr. Rath's Cellular Health Recommendations Can Help Patients With Lupus Erythematosus

Lupus erythematosus is a so-called "autoimmune" disease. It can lead to the inflammation, hardening and, eventually, failure of many organs in the body. Conventional medicine has no therapy for this serious health problem.

---

*Dear Dr. Rath:*

*I was very impressed with your research, and I was particularly interested in your theory of many degenerative diseases being related to long-term nutritional deficiencies because **my sister suffered so much from lupus erythematosus disease.** She was diagnosed with it in 1973, and since that time she has been hospitalized more times than I can remember, and has **suffered from phlebitis (inflammation of the veins) shingles, ulcerative colitis (inflammation of the bowel), and her vision has steadily deteriorated.***

*She is 44 years old, married and the mother of 3 children. In 1989, a routine pap smear showed severe inflammation and precancerous tissue. Her doctors tried to treat this condition with drugs first and later with "laser burn" treatments. This reduced the number of cells somewhat, but did not end the problem. A subsequent pap smear showed that the number of cells was increasing, and they performed a complete hysterectomy. **Even after the hysterectomy, she still had severe inflammation and a large number of pre-cancerous cells.***

***Other treatments had been also ineffective. Basically, her doctors didn't know what else to try.***

*- 1 -*

*(cont. on page 206)*

---

*(cont. from page 205)*

- 2 -

**In November of 1994, she began following your vitamin pro-gram along with a fiber drink.** *Even though she was somewhat skeptical, she felt that she had nothing to lose. In July of 1995 (after 8 months on your program), she had another pap smear test taken. What a tremendous feeling of joy she must have felt when her doctor told her that her smear came back **perfectly nor-mal with no inflammation and no pre-cancerous cells.** Her doc-tor asked her what she was doing differently, and she told her doctor about the vitamin program. Her doctor replied she didn't understand it, but couldn't argue with success.*

*There was also other benefit. In July 1995, her ophthalmologist examined her eyes. The first thing he asked was, "What have you been doing differently since your previous checkup?"* **He said her eyes were "healthier" inside than he had ever seen them during the two and a half years he'd been treating her.**

*Also, my sister is now able to limit her prednisone (anti-inflamma-tory medication) to the smallest dosage in the last 22 years. Thank you for your research and for your efforts to spread the word about breakthrough discovery.*

*Sincerely,*
*S.S.*

# Notes

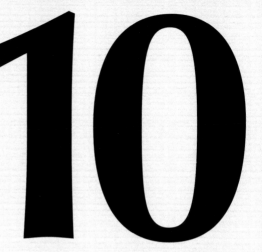

# 10

# Cellular Medicine

**Scientific Basis of Dr. Rath's Cellular Health Recommendations**

- Cellular Health Depends on Cellular Bioenergy

- The Principles of Cellular Medicine

- Scientific Facts About Cellular Nutrients

- Conventional Medicine vs. Cellular Medicine

- Questions and Answers

# Cellular Health Depends on Cellular Bioenergy

Life depends on a constant supply of four main elements: air (oxygen), water, macronutrients (proteins, fats and carbohydrates) and micronutrients (vitamins, minerals, certain amino acids and trace elements).

There is a distinct characteristic that sets micronutrients apart from air, water and food: a lack of micronutrients does not give any early "alarm" signs. Oxygen deficiency, for example, leads within minutes to the alarm suffocation. Water deficiency's alarm sign is thirst. Lack of food causes hunger.

In contrast, a deficiency of vitamins and other essential nutrients, the carriers of cellular bioenergy, do not give any alarm signs in the body. The first sign of micronutrient deficiency is the outbreak of a disease. A total depletion of vitamins, such as that in scurvy, leads to death within months. Since we all get small amounts of vitamins and other essential nutrients, we generally do not suffer from a total depletion.

Most of us, however, suffer from a chronic deficiency of vitamins and other essential nutrients over many years and decades. This long-term deficiency of cellular bioenergy is the precondition for the development of chronic diseases, such as atherosclerosis, heart failure, diabetic circulatory problems and other health conditions described in this book. The first sign of chronic micronutrient deficiency can be a heart attack, a stroke or the outbreak of disease.

Since our bodies do not give us any alarm signs, the best way we can avoid deficiencies in cellular energy — and prevent the onset of many diseases — is with optimum daily supplementation of essential nutrients contained in my Cellular Health recommendations.

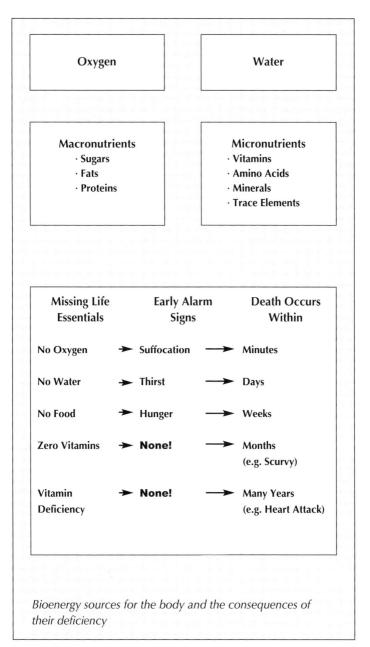

| Oxygen | Water |

| **Macronutrients** | **Micronutrients** |
| · Sugars | · Vitamins |
| · Fats | · Amino Acids |
| · Proteins | · Minerals |
| | · Trace Elements |

| Missing Life Essentials | Early Alarm Signs | Death Occurs Within |
|---|---|---|
| No Oxygen | Suffocation | Minutes |
| No Water | Thirst | Days |
| No Food | Hunger | Weeks |
| Zero Vitamins | **None!** | Months (e.g. Scurvy) |
| Vitamin Deficiency | **None!** | Many Years (e.g. Heart Attack) |

*Bioenergy sources for the body and the consequences of their deficiency*

# Cellular Medicine

This book introduces the scientific concept of Cellular Medicine, which marks a new era in health care. It is based on a new understanding of health and disease: Health and disease in our bodies and organs are determined by the functioning of millions of cells. Optimum cell functioning is a precondition for health. In contrast, cellular malfunction causes disease.

The primary, and by far the most frequent, cause of the malfunctioning of cells is a chronic deficiency of essential cellular nutrients, particularly, vitamins, amino acids, minerals and trace elements. These cellular nutrients are needed for a multitude of biochemical reactions and other cellular functions taking place in every single cell of our bodies. Chronic deficiencies of one or more of these essential nutrients, therefore, must lead to cellular malfunctioning and disease.

Cellular Medicine can also explain why cardiovascular disease is the number one cause of death in many countries. The circulatory system is mechanically the most active organ in our bodies because of the continuous pumping function of the heart and pulsatile blood flow through the arteries. Because of this high mechanical stress, the cells of the cardiovascular system have a high rate of consumption of vitamins and other essential nutrients.

Cellular Medicine defines an optimum daily intake of specific micronutrients as a basic preventive and therapeutic measure for cardiovascular disease, as well as for many other health conditions.

# The Principles of Cellular Medicine

I.  Health and disease are determined on the level of millions of cells, which compose our bodies and organs.

II. Vitamins and other essential nutrients are needed for thousands of biochemical reactions taking place in each cell. Chronic deficiency of these vitamins and other essential nutrients is the most frequent cause of malfunction of millions of body cells and the primary cause of cardiovascular disease and other chronic health conditions.

III. Cardiovascular diseases are the most prevalent diseases because cardiovascular cells consume vitamins and other essential nutrients at a high rate due to the mechanical stress on the heart and the blood vessel wall from the heartbeat and pulse wave.

IV. Optimum dietary supplementation of vitamins and other essential nutrients is the key to the prevention and effective treatment of cardiovascular disease, as well as other chronic health conditions.

# Cellular Nutrients Deliver Essential Bioenergy to Cellular "Power Plants"

Most cellular nutrients target the "power plant" in each cell. There, they help to "ignite" the biological "burning" of energy derived from sugars, proteins and fats. Compared to a conventional power plant, macronutrients are the coal and micronutrients are the ignitors of the energy-generating process. The adjacent graphic summarizes these important facts:

- **Acetyl-Coenzyme A (Acetyl-CoA),** the central molecule of cellular metabolism, is indispensable for processing all components of food (carbohydrates, proteins, fats) and their conversion into bioenergy. Vitamin B5 (pantothenic acid) is a structural component of this key molecule. A deficiency of vitamin B5 leads to decreased acetyl-coenzyme A levels and metabolic "congestion." This can result in increased blood levels of cholesterol and other blood fats. Optimum supplementation of vitamin B5 corrects this "congestion" and improves the production of cellular energy.

- **Vitamin B3 (nicotinic acid)** is the energy transport molecule of one of the most important cellular energy carriers, nicotinamide adenine dinucleotide (NAD). Vitamin C provides the bioenergy to NAD transport molecules by adding hydrogen atoms (-H) and thus, biological energy. The energy-rich shuttle molecules NAD-H provide energy for thousands of cellular reactions. A sufficient supply of vitamin B3 and vitamin C is indispensable for optimum cellular energy.

- **Vitamin B2 (riboflavin)** and vitamin C cooperate in a similar way within each cell as a bioenergy shuttle. Vitamin B2 is a structural component of the energy transport molecule flavin adenine dinucleotide (FAD), and vitamin C provides bioenergy for the activation of millions of bioenergy-rich FAD molecules.

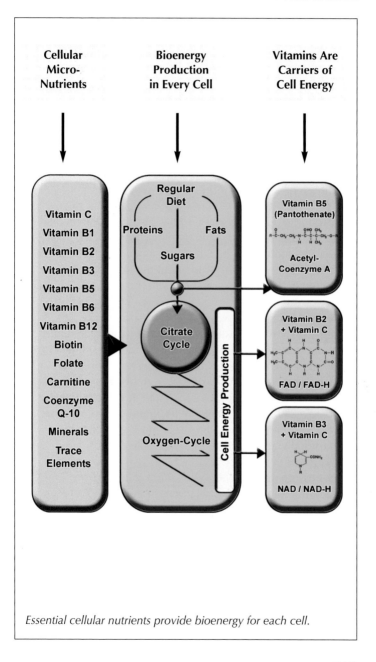

**Cellular Micro-Nutrients**

Vitamin C
Vitamin B1
Vitamin B2
Vitamin B3
Vitamin B5
Vitamin B6
Vitamin B12
Biotin
Folate
Carnitine
Coenzyme Q-10
Minerals
Trace Elements

**Bioenergy Production in Every Cell**

Regular Diet

Proteins     Fats

Sugars

Citrate Cycle

Oxygen-Cycle

Cell Energy Production

**Vitamins Are Carriers of Cell Energy**

Vitamin B5 (Pantothenate)

Acetyl-Coenzyme A

Vitamin B2 + Vitamin C

FAD / FAD-H

Vitamin B3 + Vitamin C

NAD / NAD-H

*Essential cellular nutrients provide bioenergy for each cell.*

215

# Scientific Facts About the Nutrients in Dr. Rath's Cellular Health Recommendations

The worldwide success of my Cellular Health recommendations is due to the fact that this natural program is scientifically based. The exact biochemical composition and many biological functions of the ingredients of these recommendations are known. Thus, the health benefits of this program are reproducible, and millions of people around the world can benefit from them now and in future generations.

For each component of my Cellular Health recommendations, there are numerous scientific studies substantiating their great importance for human health. The following pages summarize the comprehensive knowledge about the importance of each of the ingredients in this essential nutrient program.

Interestingly, many of these biochemical functions are already contained in leading textbooks of biology and biochemistry. In sharp contrast, many textbooks in medicine are still lacking this lifesaving knowledge. The leading textbook for cardiologists, Eugene Braunwald's *Heart Disease – A Textbook of Cardiovascular Medicine,* does not mention vitamin C one single time in 2,000 pages of teaching material for future cardiologists, despite the fact that this vitamin is the single most important reason why animals don't get heart attacks, but people do.

The omission of this lifesaving information in medical textbooks is no coincidence. It happens in the interest of the multitrillion dollar pharmaceutical investment "business with disease." This investment industry is based on patented, synthetic drugs that merely target symptoms. The continuation and global expansion of this industry depends on eliminating any competition from natural, non-patentable approaches to health. Preventing doctors and other health professionals from recognizing the role of micronutrients as the basis for optimum cellular function and human health serves this goal.

The scientific basis of Cellular Medicine can bring about the necessary and long overdue modernization of medicine. Each day that the implementation of Cellular Medicine is delayed, thousands of patients worldwide will continue to die from preventable diseases.

The following pages contain the most important scientific facts about the components of my Cellular Health recommendations. This information will also help an increasing number of physicians and health professionals accept and implement the principles of Cellular Medicine in their daily practices.

# Vitamins, Minerals, Trace Elements, Amino Acids and Other Cellular Nutrients

### Vitamin C
Vitamin C is the key nutrient for the stability of our blood vessels, our hearts, and all other organs in our bodies. Without vitamin C, our bodies would literally collapse and dissolve, as in scurvy. Vitamin C is responsible for the optimum production and function of collagen, elastin and other connective tissue molecules that give stability to our blood vessels and our entire bodies.

Vitamin C is important for fast wound healing throughout our bodies, including the healing of millions of tiny wounds and lesions inside our blood vessel walls.

Vitamin C is the most important antioxidant in the body. Optimum amounts of vitamin C effectively protect the cardiovascular system and body against biological rusting.

Vitamin C is also a cofactor for a series of biological catalysts (enzymes), which are important for the improved metabolism of cholesterol, triglycerides and other risk factors. This helps to decrease the risk for cardiovascular disease.

Vitamin C is an important energy molecule needed to recharge energy carriers inside the cells.

217

## Vitamin E

Vitamin E is the most important fat-soluble antioxidant vitamin. It protects, particularly, the membranes of the cells in our cardiovascular systems. Vitamin E also prevents free radical attacks and oxidative damage.

Vitamin E is carried in low-density lipoproteins (LDL) and other cholesterol and fat-transporting particles. Taken in optimum amounts, vitamin E can prevent these fat particles from oxidizing (biological rusting) and damaging the inside of blood vessel walls.

Vitamin E was shown to render the platelets in blood circulation less sticky and, thereby, keep the blood thin and decrease the risk of blood clotting.

## Beta-carotene

Beta-carotene is also called pro-vitamin A, and is another important fat-soluble antioxidant vitamin. Like vitamin E, it is transported primarily in lipoprotein particles in the bloodstream to millions of body cells. Also like vitamin E, beta-carotene prevents these fat particles from rusting and damaging the cardiovascular system. Beta-carotene is documented in a rapidly growing number of clinical studies as another protective agent against cardiovascular disease. Similar to vitamin E, beta-carotene has been shown to decrease the risk of blood clotting.

## Vitamin B1 (Thiamine)

Thiamine functions as the cofactor of an important biocatalyst called pyrophosphate. This catalyst is involved in phosphate metabolism in our cells, another key energy source that optimizes millions of reactions in cardiovascular and other cells.

## Vitamin B2 (Riboflavin)

Riboflavin is the cofactor for flavin adenine dinucleotide (FAD), one of the most important carrier molecules of cellular energy inside the tiny energy centers (power plants) of all cells.

## Vitamin B3 (Niacin, Niacinamide)

Niacin is an important nutrient, essential as the cofactor of nicotinamide adenine dinucleotide (NAD) and related energy carrier molecules. This energy carrier molecule is one of the most important energy transport systems in the entire body. Millions of these carriers are created and recharged (by vitamin C) inside the cellular energy centers of the cardiovascular system and the body. Cell life, and life in general, would not be possible without this energy carrier.

## Vitamin B5 (Pantothenate)

Pantothenate is the cofactor of coenzyme A, the central fuel molecule in the metabolism of our heart cells, blood vessel cells and all other cells. The metabolism of carbohydrates, proteins and fats inside each cell all lead to a single molecule, acetyl-coenzyme A. This molecule is the key molecule that helps to convert all food into cell energy. This important molecule is actually composed, in part, of vitamin B5 and the importance of supplementing this vitamin is evident. Again, cell life would not be possible without this vitamin.

## Vitamin B6 (Pyridoxine)

Vitamin B6 is the cofactor of pyridoxal phosphate, an important cofactor for the metabolism of amino acids and proteins in cardiovascular and other cells. Vitamin B6 is needed for the production of red blood cells, which are the carriers of oxygen to the cells of the cardiovascular system and all other cells in the body. Vitamin B6 is also essential for the optimum structure and function of collagen fibers.

## Vitamin B12

Vitamin B12 is needed for the proper metabolism of fatty acids and certain amino acids in the cells of our bodies. Vitamin B12 is also required for the production of red blood cells. A severe deficiency of vitamin B12 can cause a disease called pernicious anemia, which is characterized by an insufficient production of blood cells.

### Folate

Folate is a very important nutrient for the production of red blood cells and oxygen supply.

The last three vitamins are good examples of how these bioenergy molecules work together in synergy, like an orchestra. Without proper oxygen transport to all the cells, their function would be impaired, no matter how much of the other vitamins you might take. It is, therefore, important to supplement your diet as completely as possible with the right essential nutrients in the right amounts.

### Biotin

Biotin is needed for the metabolism of carbohydrates, fats and proteins.

### Vitamin D

Vitamin D is essential for optimum calcium and phosphate metabolism in the body. Vitamin D is needed for the growth and stability of the bones and teeth. For centuries, vitamin D deficiency was a frequent children's condition, causing retarded growth and malformation. Thus, in many countries, milk is enriched with vitamin D.

Vitamin D is also essential for optimum calcium metabolism in the artery walls, including the removal of calcium from atherosclerotic deposits.

## Minerals

Minerals are important essential nutrients. Calcium, magnesium and potassium are the most important among them. Minerals are needed for a multitude of catalytic reactions occurring in each cell in the body.

## Calcium

Calcium is important for the proper contraction of muscle cells, including millions of heart muscle cells. It is needed for the conduction of nerve impulses and, therefore, for optimum heartbeat. Calcium is also essential for the hardening and stability of our bones and teeth. It is also needed for the proper biological communication among the cells of the cardiovascular system and most other cells, as well as for many other biological functions.

## Magnesium

Magnesium is nature's calcium antagonist, and its benefit for the cardiovascular system is similar to the calcium antagonist drugs that are prescribed, except that magnesium is produced by nature itself.

Clinical studies have shown that magnesium is particularly important for helping to normalize elevated blood pressure; moreover, it can help normalize irregular heartbeat.

# Trace Elements

The trace elements zinc, manganese, copper, selenium, chromium and molybdenum are also important essential nutrients. Most of the trace elements are metals needed as catalysts for thousands of biochemical reactions in the metabolism of cells. However, they are needed only in very tiny amounts – less than one tenth of a thousandth of a gram.

# Amino Acids

Amino acids are the building blocks of proteins. Most of the amino acids in our bodies are derived from regular food and from digesting proteins. Many amino acids can be synthesized in our bodies when needed; these amino acids are called "non-essential" amino acids. Those amino acids that the body *cannot* synthesize are called "essential" amino acids.

It is important to understand that — even though the body can produce certain amino acids — the amount produced may not be enough to maintain proper health. A good example is the amino acid proline.

### Proline

The amino acid proline is a major building block of the stability proteins collagen and elastin. More than 10% of the building blocks of collagen molecules consist of proline alone. It is easy to understand how important it is for the optimum stability of our blood vessels, and our bodies in general, to get an optimum amount of proline in our diets.

Proline is very important in the process of reversing atherosclerotic deposits. As described in this book, cholesterol-carrying fat globules (lipoproteins) attach to the inside of the blood vessel wall via biological adhesive tapes. Proline is a formidable "Teflon" agent, which can neutralize the stickiness of these fat globules. The therapeutic effect is twofold. First, proline helps to prevent the further buildup of atherosclerotic deposits and second, proline helps to release already deposited fat globules from the blood vessel wall into the bloodstream. When many fat globules are released from the plaques in the artery walls, the deposit size decreases and leads to a reversal of cardiovascular disease.

Proline can be synthesized by the body, but the amounts synthesized are frequently inadequate, particularly in patients with an increased risk for cardiovascular disease.

## Lysine

As opposed to proline, lysine is an essential amino acid, which means that the body cannot synthesize it. Daily supplementation of this amino acid is, therefore, critical. Lysine, like proline, is an important building block of collagen and other stability molecules, and its intake helps to stabilize the blood vessels and other organs in the body.

The combined intake of lysine and proline with vitamin C is of particular importance for the optimum stability of body tissue. For optimum strength of the collagen molecules, its building blocks lysine and proline need to be biochemically modified to hydroxy lysine and hydroxy proline. Vitamin C is the most effective biocatalyst for accomplishing this "hydroxylation" reaction and, thereby, for providing optimum strength to the connective tissue.

Lysine is another "Teflon" agent, which can help release deposited fat globules from the blood vessel deposits. People with existing cardiovascular disease may increase their daily intake of lysine and proline to several grams in addition to the basic program recommended in this book.

Lysine is also the precursor for the amino acid carnitine. The conversion of lysine into carnitine requires the presence of vitamin C as a biocatalyst. This is another reason why the combination of lysine and vitamin C is essential.

## Arginine

Arginine has many functions in the human body. In connection with the cardiovascular system, one function is of particular importance. The amino acid arginine can split off a small molecule called nitric oxide. This tiny part of the former arginine molecule has a powerful role in maintaining cardiovascular health. Nitric oxide relaxes the blood vessel walls and helps to normalize high blood pressure. In addition, nitric oxide helps to decrease the stickiness of platelets and has an anti-clogging effect.

## Carnitine

Carnitine is a very important essential nutrient. It is needed for the conversion of fat into energy. Carnitine functions like a shuttle between the cell factory and the energy compartment within each cell. It transports energy molecules in and out of these cellular power plants. This mechanism is particularly important for all muscle cells, including those of the heart.

For the constantly pumping heart muscle, carnitine is one of the most critical "cell fuels." Thus, it is not surprising that many clinical studies have documented the great value of carnitine supplementation in improving the pumping function and performance of the heart.

Carnitine also benefits the electrical cells of the heart, and its supplementation has been shown to help normalize different forms of irregular heartbeat.

## Cysteine

Cysteine is another important amino acid with many important functions in the body. The cardiovascular system benefits particularly from supplementation with this amino acid because cysteine is a building block of glutathione, one of the most important antioxidants produced in the body. Among other functions, glutathione protects the inside of blood vessel walls from free radical and other kinds of damage.

# Other Important Cellular Nutrients

### Coenzyme Q-10

Coenzyme Q-10 is another important essential nutrient. It is also known as ubiquinone. Coenzyme Q-10 functions as an extremely important catalyst for the energy center of each cell. Because of its high workload, the heart muscle cells have a particularly high demand for coenzyme Q-10. In patients with insufficient pumping function of the heart, this essential nutrient is frequently deficient. An irrefutable number of clinical studies have documented the great value of coenzyme Q-10 in treating heart failure and optimizing heart performance.

## Inositol

Inositol is a component of lecithin. It is essential for sugar and fat metabolism in the cells of our bodies.

Inositol is also important for the biological communication process between the cells and organs in the body. Hormones, such as insulin and other molecules, are signals from outside the cell. If a hormone docks to a cell, it needs to transmit information to that cell. Inositol is part of the proper reading mechanism of this information through the cell membrane. Thus, inositol is part of the proper biological communication process, which in turn, is critical for optimum cardiovascular health.

## Pycnogenols and Other Bioflavonoids

Pycnogenols refers to a group of bioflavonoids (pro-anthocyanidins) with remarkable properties. In the cardiovascular system, pycnogenols have several important functions:

- Pycnogenols are powerful antioxidants that work together with vitamin C and vitamin E in preventing damage to the cardiovascular system by free radicals.

- Together with vitamin C, pycnogenols have a particular value in stabilizing the blood vessel walls and capillaries. Pycnogenols have been shown to bind to elastin, the most important elasticity molecule, and protect elastin molecules against enzymatic degradation.

225

# Conventional Medicine vs. Cellular Medicine:

## Conventional Medicine

My Cellular Health recommendations withstand any comparison to other preventive cardiovascular approaches. Preventive approaches by conventional medicine focus on cholesterol lowering and the reduction of other risk factors, as well as lifestyle changes. These approaches miss key targets of cardiovascular health, such as optimum vascular stability and repair, antioxidant protection and bioenergy for cells.

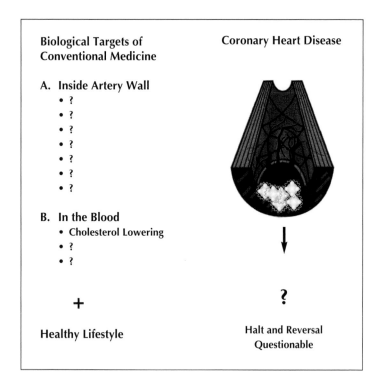

**Biological Targets of Conventional Medicine**

**Coronary Heart Disease**

**A. Inside Artery Wall**
- ?
- ?
- ?
- ?
- ?
- ?
- ?

**B. In the Blood**
- **Cholesterol Lowering**
- ?
- ?

**+**

**Healthy Lifestyle**

**?**

**Halt and Reversal Questionable**

# Comparing Therapeutic Targets in Cardiovascular Disease

## Cellular Medicine

In contrast, my Cellular Health recommendations have defined biological targets. The scientific basis of Cellular Medicine defines therapeutic targets of unprecedented scope and specificity to prevent and treat cardiovascular disease. Vascular wall stability is optimized, vascular healing processes are induced and antioxidant and "Teflon" protection is provided. The most important biological targets of this natural cardiovascular health program are summarized in the figure below.

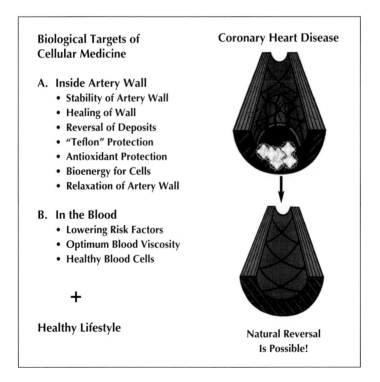

**Biological Targets of Cellular Medicine**

**Coronary Heart Disease**

A.  **Inside Artery Wall**
   - Stability of Artery Wall
   - Healing of Wall
   - Reversal of Deposits
   - "Teflon" Protection
   - Antioxidant Protection
   - Bioenergy for Cells
   - Relaxation of Artery Wall

B.  **In the Blood**
   - Lowering Risk Factors
   - Optimum Blood Viscosity
   - Healthy Blood Cells

**+**

**Healthy Lifestyle**

**Natural Reversal Is Possible!**

227

# Conventional Medicine vs. Cellular Medicine:

## Effectiveness

Conventional therapy is generally limited to the treatment of cardiovascular *symptoms,* one at a time. Since most heart disease patients have many cardiovascular problems at the same time, they frequently are prescribed several medications.

In contrast, my Cellular Health recommendations correct the underlying causes of the disease. It provides "cell fuel" for millions of cells, allowing for the correction of impaired cellular function in different compartments of the cardiovascular system simultaneously.

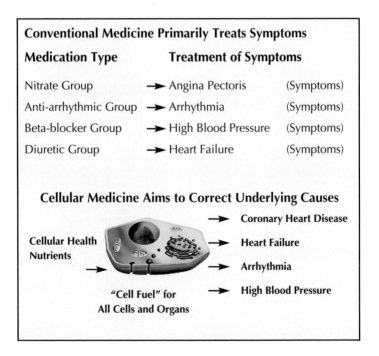

**Conventional Medicine Primarily Treats Symptoms**

| Medication Type | Treatment of Symptoms | |
|---|---|---|
| Nitrate Group | → Angina Pectoris | (Symptoms) |
| Anti-arrhythmic Group | → Arrhythmia | (Symptoms) |
| Beta-blocker Group | → High Blood Pressure | (Symptoms) |
| Diuretic Group | → Heart Failure | (Symptoms) |

**Cellular Medicine Aims to Correct Underlying Causes**

Cellular Health Nutrients

→ Coronary Heart Disease
→ Heart Failure
→ Arrhythmia
→ High Blood Pressure

"Cell Fuel" for All Cells and Organs

# Comparing Effectiveness and Safety

## Safety

Another important advantage of my Cellular Health recommendations compared to conventional drug therapies is that they are safe and undesirable side effects are unknown. Dr. A. Bendich summarized the safety aspects of vitamins in a review in the *New York Academy of Sciences*. She found that all rumors about the side effects of vitamins are unsubstantiated. These deceptions are being spread in the interest of the pharmaceutical industry to create a false dependency on prescription drugs alone.

Below, my Cellular Health recommendations are compared to conventional cardiovascular therapies and their risks.

### Conventional Medicine

| Therapy | Potential Side Effects | References |
|---|---|---|
| Cholesterol-lowering Drugs | Cancer, Liver Damage and Myopathy (Muscle Weakness) | Physician's Desk Reference (PDR) |
| Aspirin | Strokes, Ulcers, Collagen Breakdown and Promotes Heart Disease | PDR Brooks |
| Calcium Channel Blockers | Cancer | Psaty |

### Cellular Medicine

| Therapy | Potential Side Effects | References |
|---|---|---|
| Essential Nutrients | None | Bendich, Rath (*Why Animals Don't Get Heart Attacks, But People Do, First Edition*) |

# How You Can Live Longer and Stay Healthy

The same biological mechanisms that lead to the hardening of arteries and cardiovascular disease determine the process of aging in your body. One could say that the aging of your body is a slow form of cardiovascular disease. The speed at which it ages is directly dependent on the state of the health of your cardiovascular system. Particularly important is the optimum functioning of the 60,000-mile-long pipeline of your arteries, veins and capillaries. This blood vessel pipeline supplies all the organs of your body and its billions of body cells with oxygen and essential nutrients.

## Your body is as old as its cardiovascular system.

If you do not protect your body with essential nutrients, the aging process leads to a gradual thickening of your blood vessel walls. This eventually leads to the malnutrition of millions of your body's cells and an accelerated aging of your entire body and its organs.

My Cellular Health recommendations are a proven way to protect your cardiovascular system. It is also the best way to help retard the aging process of your body in a natural way and, thereby, contribute to a long and healthy life.

# Questions and Answers About Dr. Rath's Cellular Health Recommendations

The following are some of the most frequently asked questions about my Cellular Health recommendations. The responses are general advice that cannot replace a personal consultation with your doctor.

### *What are Dr. Rath's Cellular Health recommendations?*

They are a daily nutrient program composed of specific vitamins, amino acids, minerals and trace elements scientifically developed to optimize the function of the cardiovascular system. My recommendations comprise a program in which the chosen ingredients work synergistically together. It is complemented by moderate lifestyle changes as outlined in the "Ten Step Program for Natural Cardiovascular Health" in the first chapter of this book.

### *What sets Dr. Rath's Cellular Health recommendations apart from other multivitamins?*

My nutrient program is based on a new and scientifically correct understanding about the causes of cardiovascular disease and other chronic health conditions. Its effectiveness has been proven in clinical studies and in hundreds of thousands of people who have used these recommendations for natural prevention and basic therapy. Their nutrient composition is carefully chosen for maximum synergy of these ingredients to achieve optimum health benefits in the millions of cells. This fact also explains why these moderately dosed nutrients are more effective than megadoses of individual ingredients recommended elsewhere.

Within only a few years, my Cellular Health recommendations have become the world's leading natural health program that is followed by hundreds of thousands of people around the world.

231

### Who can benefit from Dr. Rath's Cellular Health recommendations?

Every man and woman, from teenager to senior citizen, can benefit from these recommendations. My *Basic* Cellular Health recommendations are primarily a preventive health program for avoiding cardiovascular disease and other health problems. Patients suffering from cardiovascular disease, high blood pressure, heart failure and other health problems should complement these *basic* recommendations with the *special* "add-on" nutrient programs developed for specific health problems described in this book.

People living with physical or emotional stress, those in cities with high air pollution and elderly people should increase their basic daily nutrient intake.

### Are there any side effects from Dr. Rath's Cellular Health recommendations?

All the components of my recommendations are nutrients, or natural substances, known to the body. Therefore, your body is able to decide how much it needs of each of these ingredients. Side effects, such as those from overdosing on pharmaceutical drugs, will not occur even if you double or triple the dosages recommended in this book.

### Should I continue my regular prescription medication when starting on Dr. Rath's Cellular Health recommendations?

Yes. If you are a patient, do not change or discontinue any prescription medication without consulting with your doctor. My nutrient programs are an adjunct to conventional therapy, not a substitute for your doctor's advice. You should also know that a growing number of doctors are already recommending my nutrient programs because they are scientifically based and clinically tested.

### Is a healthy lifestyle more important than taking vitamins?

This is a misconception that needs to be clarified. The bioenergy components of my Cellular Health recommendations are the basis for any successful prevention and treatment of cardio-vascular conditions. As explained in detail throughout this book, cardiovascular disease develops because the cardiovascular cells are depleted of vitamins and other bioenergy fuel. Refilling this bioenergy is, therefore, the basic preventive and therapeutic measure for cardiovascular health. Lifestyle changes can add to these biological measures, but they are not able to replace them.

### *What about natural cardiovascular programs based on heavy exercise, yoga or oriental philosophies?*

Any cardiovascular health recommendation that does not include refilling the cells with essential vitamins and other micronutrients creates false hope. In fact, these programs are outright dangerous. No heart patient has to become a fakir, triathlete or yoga master to optimize cardiovascular health. Moreover, a strict diet further aggravates the deficiencies of essential nutrients. For example, the artery "Teflon" amino acids lysine and proline are primarily found in meat products. Don't be confused by self-appointed diet apostles and yoga masters. Vitamins and other sources of cellular bioenergy remain the basis of natural cardiovascular health.

### *When can a patient expect health improvements when following Dr. Rath's Cellular Health recommendations?*

Every human being is different, and the time it takes before health improvements are noticeable cannot be generalized. Patients with elevated blood pressure, irregular heartbeat or shortness of breath, for example, may experience health improvements in the relatively short time of a few weeks. In contrast, the healing process of the artery walls and the reversal of atherosclerosis is a long-term process that requires months or years.

Once your health has improved, you should be sure to continue to follow my Cellular Health recommendations to minimize the risk of the recurrence of any health problems.

233

# Notes

# 11

# Eradicating
# Heart Disease

- Why You May Not Have Heard About
  This Medical Breakthrough Before

- The Ten Laws of the Pharmaceutical Industry

- Key Tricks of the "Business With Disease"

- A New Era of Human Health Begins

- Milestones Towards Eradicating Heart Disease

- Principles of a New Health Care System

# Why You May Not Have Heard About This Medical Breakthrough Before

As you have read about the remarkable health benefits of vitamins throughout this book, you may have asked yourself: "Why is this lifesaving information not used by every doctor and in every hospital? Why is the information that animals don't get heart attacks because they produce their own vitamin C not covered on every TV and radio channel and on the front pages of newspapers? Why did we not learn about this in kindergarten?"

There is an entire industry with an innate economic interest to obstruct, suppress and discredit any information about the natural eradication of diseases. The pharmaceutical industry makes over one trillion dollars from selling drugs for ongoing diseases. These drugs may relieve symptoms, but they do not cure. We have to realize that the mission of this industry is to make money from *ongoing* diseases. The cure or eradication of a disease will lead to the collapse of the trillion dollar market of pharmaceuticals.

I encourage you to read the following key points about the nature of the pharmaceutical industry and think about each of them. Now you will understand why we are bombarded with advertising campaigns by pharmaceutical companies wanting to make us believe that they are "searching for cures," "striving for the eradication of diseases," "increasing life expectancy" and other false promises.

With these deceptive statements, the pharmaceutical industry has for decades been able to disguise the true nature of its business – maximum profit from ongoing diseases.

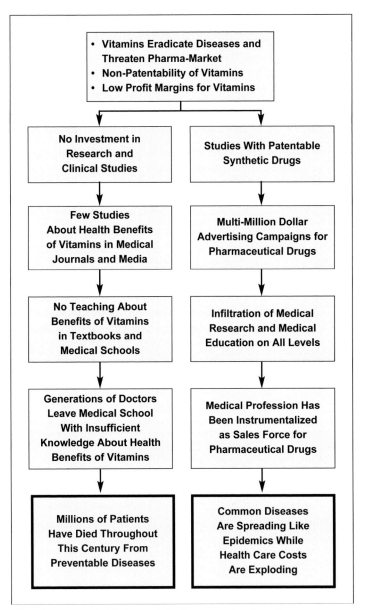

*The pharmaceutical industry is built on two deadly columns.*

# The Ten Laws of the Pharmaceutical Industry

Until now, the pharmaceutical industry has presented itself as a benefactor to mankind that no modern society could exist without. A simple analysis of the nature of the pharmaceutical industry, however, reveals a realistic picture, which can be summarized as follows:

**1**     **The pharmaceutical industry is not a naturally grown health industry, but an artificially created investment business based on the deceptive promise to deliver health.**

**2**     **The marketplace of the pharmaceutical industry is your body — but only as long as it is sick.**

**3**     **Prevention, root cause treatment and, above all, eradication of diseases decrease or destroy the pharmaceutical markets and are, therefore, not in the interest of this industry.**

**4**     **The great majority of pharmaceutical drugs have no proven efficacy and are merely symptom oriented.**

**5**     **The basis of the enormous profits of this industry is not effectively fighting diseases, but the patent royalties of newly synthesized molecules unknown to the human body.**

**6**     **Because most pharmaceutical drugs are synthetic molecules, they are toxic to the human body and frequently cause serious side effects, new diseases or even death.**

**7**  To hide this global deception scheme, the pharmaceutical industry spends more money to disguise its deceptive business scheme than for research. This money is used for thorough advertising, lobbying and other measures.

**8**  Vitamins and other natural health therapies are threatening the very basis of the pharmaceutical business for two reasons: First, they prevent or treat the root cause of today's most common diseases. Second, they are generally not patentable and therefore have low profit margins.

**9**  Natural health therapies and the pharmaceutical "business with disease" are incompatible and cannot coexist.

**10**  The precondition for the long-term prosperity of the pharmaceutical industry is the elimination of natural therapies.

---

The health and lives of hundreds of millions of people and the economies of all countries are held hostage by the pharmaceutical investment "business with disease."

Pharmaceutical companies spend twice the amount of money on marketing drugs than they do on actual research. Deceptive advertising campaigns, such as the one depicted here, give millions false hope.

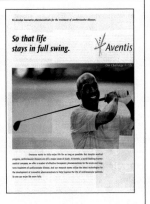

239

# Key Tricks of the Pharmaceutical "Business With Disease"

For more than a century, the efforts of the pharmaceutical investment industry to replace natural non-patentable therapies was strategically organized with one goal only: to establish a monopoly of pharmaceutical drugs over global health.

The unscrupulous tricks the pharmaceutical industry has used to deceive the public and establish its control can be summarized in three unscrupulous tactics:

**1** **Keeping You Uninformed:** Nearly 100 years after Dr. Szent-Gyoergy discovered the vitamin C molecule, few people know that the human body does not produce its own vitamin C. Now, it turns out that vitamin C is the single most important molecule for stabilizing the blood vessel walls and preventing cardiovascular disease.

Do you think that this health illiteracy is a coincidence? Can you believe that you, your parents and your grandparents were kept in "the dark" on purpose? Can you believe that there was a special interest group — the pharmaceutical industry — that knowingly watched cardiovascular disease develop into an epidemic during the 20th century? Can you believe that they did this for financial greed and to create a multi-billion dollar market for beta-blockers, calcium blockers and other symptom-oriented cardiovascular drugs? You better belief it.

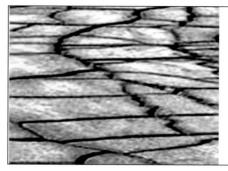

*Without the knowledge that we humans cannot produce vitamin C, our bodies become like a desert. The pharmaceutical industry had the water, but did not give it to us because they made money from selling "droplets."*

**2** Discrediting Vitamins and Natural Therapies: Whenever the truth about the health benefits of natural therapies spreads and starts to threaten the pharmaceutical investment "business with disease," the pharma-cartel launches a global scare campaign with the goal of discrediting natural, non-patentable therapies. Over the years, these deceptive PR campaigns included false information about alleged vitamin side effects ranging from cancer to mental disorders. If even one of these "pharma fairy tales" were true, we would be rather alone on Planet Earth: most other living beings would have been extinct long ago because they produce high amounts of vitamin C in their own bodies while enjoying excellent health.

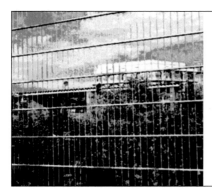

*The pharma-cartel hides its protectionist plans under the cover of "consumer protection." For years, the pharma-cartel held meetings at the Federal Ministry for Consumer Protection in Berlin, Germany in order to push their global agenda.*
Note: *The cartel has to be protected from consumers by barbed wire!*

**3** Banning Natural Health Therapies by Law: Whenever the truth about the health benefits of natural therapies spreads even further, the pharma-cartel pulls out the next measure to block it. Through their political lobbyists, they influence and abuse the political institutions in essentially all countries of the world. They have pushed legislation restricting access to natural health therapies through the European Commission (cabinet). By abusing the United Nation's "Codex Alimentarius Commission," the pharma-cartel is striving to outlaw the dissemination of natural therapies worldwide — a global protectionist law in the interest of pharmaceutical globalization.

# Deception Is a Precondition for the Pharmaceutical "Business With Disease"

How is it that millions of people are still willing to pay billions of dollars for drugs that do not cure and frequently harm?

Over the past century, the pharma-cartel and its army of lobbyists have infiltrated all sectors of our society. They have strategically built an intricate maze of manipulation, deception and control. The most important elements of this scheme are summarized on the opposite page:

- **Manipulation** of research so that synthetic drugs rather than natural therapies appear as "medicine."

- **Endorsement** of the pharmaceutical "business with disease" by doctors and other health professionals recommending ineffective drugs. Many of them are "victims" themselves because they have been deprived of adequate training in nutritional medicine during their medical education.

- **Deception** by multi-million dollar advertising campaigns on television and in other mass media that deceive the public about the efficacy and risks of pharmaceutical drugs.

- **Regulation and legislation** brought about by regulatory agencies and politicians under the pressure of an army of pharmaceutical lobbyists.

In the future, no nation will be able to afford to burden its economy with a pharmaceutical industry that grows like a cancer at the expense of people, corporations and the public sector. All these groups are suffocating from exploding health care costs for  medicines that do not cure.

The book that you hold in your hands will change that forever.

242

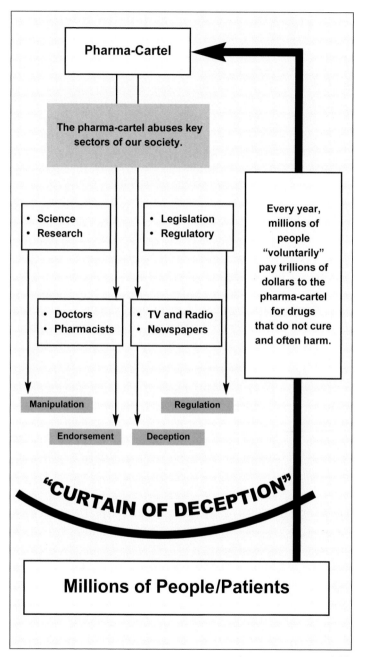

# A New Era of Human Health Begins

Five hundred years ago, the Medieval Church made billions of Thaler (early dollars) by selling indulgences, an imaginary "key to heaven," to its believers. Then, the fraud scheme collapsed and with it, much of the power of the church. Today, the pharma-business uses the same fraud scheme. It tries to sell the "key to health" to millions of people and takes away trillions of dollars in return for an illusion: the deception that the pharmaceutical industry is interested in your health.

Considering this unhealthy state of affairs, the urgency for a new health care system is obvious. The liberation from the yoke of the pharmaceutical industry will immediately and directly benefit millions of people, the business community and the public sector of all nations. This new health care system is based on the improved knowledge and participation of millions of people. Basic health has become understandable, doable and affordable for everyone. The era in human history when health was delegated to an industry that shamelessly took advantage of it is over and gone.

The new health care system focuses on primary health care, prevention and eradication of diseases. Health consultants and health centers will replace many of the medical high-tech centers of today. *Every person has the chance to become an Architect and every living room can become a consulting center of a new Health Care System.*

The new health care system is being built by dedicated laypeople, together with a growing number of doctors and health professionals. The majority of health professionals have realized that they themselves have been compromised by pharmaceutical companies and have become victims of drug-centered health care.

244

# Milestones on the Way to Eradicating Heart Disease

In this chapter, I would like to share with you an account of this advance in cardiovascular health, the milestones we have already passed, the obstacles we have overcome and the breathtaking perspective of the improvement of human health on a global level.

## The Background

In 1990, I came to America with a discovery in my suitcase that would lead to a new scientific rationale in cardiovascular disease. The message was clear: vitamins are the key to the control of cardiovascular disease, the number one killer in the industrialized world. But this breakthrough was not immediately embraced. When I decided to give up my clinical career to pursue this research avenue, many of my colleagues in Germany warned me that working on vitamins would ruin my career.

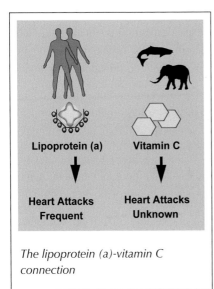

*The lipoprotein (a)-vitamin C connection*

During 1989, I presented lectures and introduced my research project to leading cardiovascular research centers in America, among them the Baylor College of Medicine in Houston, the University of Chicago, the National Institutes of Health and the University of California at La Jolla. Everywhere, the new risk factor lipoprotein (a) was met with great interest, but work on vitamins was still considered too

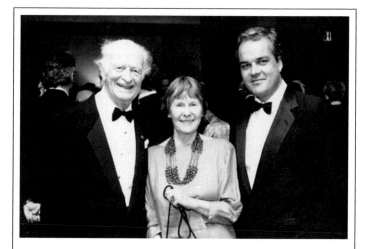

*My cooperation and friendship with two-time Nobel Laureate Linus Pauling (left) was so close that Pauling asked me (right) to continue his life work. In the center is Dr. Pauling's then-secretary Dorothy Munro.*

controversial. In early 1990, I accepted the invitation of Dr. Linus Pauling to work with him, only to discover that at age 89 he had become tired of fighting and a breakthrough for vitamins in medicine was nowhere in sight. Heartened by my discoveries, Pauling and I founded two companies in order to jump-start this process.

1990 was also the year when America's worst prescription drug disaster came to light. An estimated 50,000 Americans had died from taking an anti-arrhythmic drug that actually caused arrest of the heartbeat and sudden cardiac death. This was the same number of people killed in the Vietnam War. A Congressional investigation established that the FDA had approved this drug without any controlled clinical studies. This tragedy is presented in Thomas Moore's book *Deadly Medicine*, a must-read for everyone. Thus, while drug research had reached another deadlock, vitamins and essential nutrients as effective and safe alternatives were still ostracized by conventional medicine and restricted by the regulatory climate.

Nutritional medicine was a "stepchild" in America, but the situation was even worse in Europe. When you wanted to ship a bottle of 1,000 mg tablets of Vitamin C to Germany, it was returned by customs because vitamin C pills above 500 mg were considered drugs. This was the state of affairs only five years ago. It is with this background that we can truly appreciate the milestones we have reached and the obstacles we have been able to remove in the meantime. In the next section of this book, I will give you an account of this process from my personal experience.

**Milestone 1: Breakthrough Discovery**

The first step toward the control of cardiovascular disease was the discovery of the connection between lipoprotein (a) and vitamin C. The human body produces the risk factor lipoprotein (a) to compensate for a lack of the body's own vitamin C production. As a result, every second human being dies from heart attacks and strokes, while cardiovascular disease is essentially unknown in the animal world. This discovery fueled my interest in vitamin research.

By 1991, the conceptual work was completed and I summarized it in two scientific articles: "Solution to the Puzzle of Human Cardiovascular Disease" and "A Unified Theory of Human Cardiovascular Disease Leading the Way to the Abolition of This Disease as a Cause of Human Mortality." These publications presented for the first time the scientific rationale that heart attacks and strokes are preventable and that cardiovascular disease can be eradicated. I cited Linus Pauling, who supported these far-reaching conclusions, as co-author.

**Milestone 2: New Understanding of the Nature of Cardiovascular Disease**

The new understanding about the nature of cardiovascular disease is presented in detail in this book. This new understanding clarifies that the primary cause of cardiovascular disease is

247

not high cholesterol or a high fat diet. These factors can only become risk factors if the wall of our arteries is already weakened by vitamin deficienc — and only then. I had identified cardiovascular disease essentially as an early form of the sailor's disease scurvy.

It also became clear that atherosclerotic plaques in our arteries are not random events; these plaques are simply a "scaffold" of nature to stabilize and repair the blood vessel walls once they have become weakened by vitamin deficiency. Finally, this new scientific rationale can also explain why we get infarctions of the heart and not of the nose or ears. Moreover, I found that most inherited disorders known today as risk factors for cardiovascular disease — including high cholesterol, triglycerides and homocysteine levels — can be ameliorated by high vitamin intake.

Obviously, a new scientific rationale that could suddenly explain so many unsolved mysteries about the number one health problem would not go unnoticed. At that time, it became clear to the pharmaceutical companies and medical opinion leaders that the cholesterol dogma and a huge prescription drug market would eventually collapse. The time this would take was dependent only on one factor: how fast the discovery of the scurvy-heart disease connection could be spread globally. Thus, it was in 1990 that a giant battle for public perception began with the trillion dollar pharmaceutical industry fighting for its survival.

But there were also other voices early on. One of the first encouraging messages came from Dr. Valentin Fuster, then head of cardiology at Harvard Medical School and later president of the American Heart Association. Already in 1992, Dr. Fuster wrote to me, "You may be quite correct in your predictions about the role of vitamin C in cardiovascular disease." He stated that his own department would start in this line of research. Unfortunately, I have not heard any results since.

## Milestone 3: Watershed Media Event

The next step in this process was the key media support for vitamins and nutritional medicine. The cover story *"The Real Power of Vitamins"* in the April 1992 issue of *TIME Magazine* was triggered by an international conference on vitamins held by the New York Academy of Sciences in February of that year. Many scientists contributed to this conference. I was privileged to be one of them, and introduced our new understanding about the nature of cardiovascular disease, including the key role of vitamins in its prevention.

After decades of bias and boycotts against vitamins in the media, this issue of *TIME Magazine* became a watershed event. Studies documenting the benefits of vitamins in the prevention of many diseases were no longer being automatically rejected. Only weeks after this *TIME Magazine* article, an important epidemiological study led by Dr. James Enstrom and his colleagues from the University of California, Los Angeles received national attention. It showed that long-term vitamin C supplementation, as opposed to the average American diet, could cut the rate for heart disease almost in half. Thus, the suddenly available and positive media coverage led to a change of perception in favor of vitamins with worldwide repercussions.

Now, more than a decade later, the "media battle" about the health benefits of vitamins is still being waged with fierce opposition organized from drug companies rapidly losing ground.

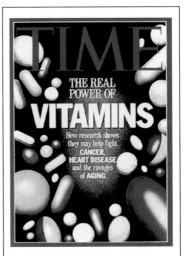

*TIME Magazine, April 1992*

249

## Milestone 4: New Legislation Guarantees Free Access to Vitamins

In retrospect, 1992 was a remarkable year. On July 2, 1992, Linus Pauling and I held a press conference in San Francisco issuing a "Call for an International Scientific Effort to Eradicate Heart Disease." Our simple but powerful message was that the scientific basis and means to eradicate heart disease — the number one cause of death in industrialized countries — were available (for details, see Chapter 12).

Only weeks after this public announcement, the FDA, heavily influenced by the pharmaceutical industry, launched another attack on vitamins. Their goal was to pass legislation that would make vitamins and other essential nutrients available by prescription only. Why did the FDA start this battle in 1991 and why was it the fiercest attack on nutritional supplements to have been waged? This book gives you the answer: If vitamins are the solution to the cardiovascular disease epidemic — a

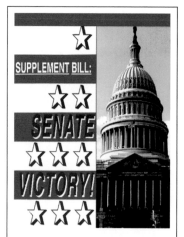

*The Dietary Supplement Health and Education Act (DSHEA)of 1994 guarantees free access to vitamins.*

prescription drug market of over hundreds of billions of dollars annually is going to collapse. But the people of America said "no" to these plans and defended their health freedom (for details, see box on page 250).

In August 1994, the U.S. Congress unanimously passed legislation preserving free access to vitamins and other essential nutrients. This victory in the battle for vitamin freedom has a truly historic dimension, and it provided an important window of opportunity to win similar battles in

# The Worst Defeat in FDA History

It is a fact that almost all "experts" at the Food and Drug Administration (FDA) have financial ties to pharmaceutical companies and are instrumentalized on behalf of the pharmaceutical industry. It was clear that millions of Americans who had been enjoying the health benefits of vitamins over decades would not understand why free access to vitamins should be restricted and why essential nutrients should become prescription items. To cover their real goal — protectionist laws for drug markets — a camouflage was used by the FDA to make these unethical plans more palatable and acceptable to the American people:

- **"Consumer Protection":** In a large-scale public relations campaign, the FDA on behalf of the pharma-cartel, tried to make millions of Americans believe that vitamins and other natural therapies had to become prescription items in order to protect them from "overdosing." The deceptive nature of this campaign was revealed when the following U.S. statistics became public: from 1983-1990, not a single person died from taking vitamins or other essential nutrients. In contrast, during the same period, hundreds of thousands of Americans had died from taking prescription drugs, which had been approved by this very same agency — the FDA!

- **"Internationalization":** The deceptive argument by which the FDA tried to restrict vitamins on behalf of the drug makers was an alleged necessity for "international trade standards." These outrageous "standards" were set by Germany and other European countries, where one gram vitamin C pills were defined as prescription drugs and amino acids were on the "black list."

Thus, on behalf of the drug industry, the FDA tried to abolish two of the most basic human rights — the right to health choices and the freedom to access health information.

But the American people were neither interested in "consumer protection" from vitamins or "internationalization" back to the "Dark Ages of Medicine." In the "largest movement since the Vietnam War" *(Newsweek),* the American people through their political representatives secured their health freedom against the FDA and the financial interests of the pharmaceutical industry.

In August 1994, the Dietary Supplement Health and Education Act (DSHEA) was passed unanimously in the Senate and House of Representatives of the U.S. Congress.

other countries and eventually, worldwide. Many contributed to this historic success, but most important were those millions of Americans who made it unmistakably clear to their political representatives that they would have free access to their vitamins today — and in the future!

The medical breakthrough in vitamin C-heart disease research that triggered this battle also helped to win it.

## Milestone 5: A Scientific Breakthrough Becomes Available for Everyone

Much of the power of this medical breakthrough comes from the fact that it has direct consequences for the health and lives of millions of people. Thus, it has to be presented in a language understandable to everyone. My popular health books — including the one you are now reading — are written so everyone can understand this medical breakthrough and immediately take advantage of it.

Why has this step been so important? One hundred years ago, when bacteria was discovered as the cause of infectious diseases, it still took several decades before the first antibiotics and vaccines were developed.

Now, with the breakthrough in cardiovascular disease, no such time is needed. Vitamins and other essential nutrients, the solution to the cardiovascular disease epidemic, are available for everyone right now. Thus, the time it will take to control this epidemic depends on one main factor: the time it will take to spread the message about the health benefits of vitamins.

My books have already empowered millions of people to take greater responsibility for their own health. They share my books not only with their family and friends, but they also discuss them with their doctors and send them to their political representatives.

Over the years, the spread of this new information has had far-reaching impacts: Major medical schools have integrated courses on nutrition in their teaching programs and nutritional medicine has become an accepted form of medicine for three out of four people. As opposed to 1992, today more people visit physicians and other health professionals who apply natural therapies than conventional physicians. These are just a few highlights documenting the dramatic transition of health care in the past decade.

## Milestone 6: Cellular Medicine — Foundation of a New Health Care System

The discovery of the nature of cardiovascular disease was just the beginning. With the course of further research, it became clear that most of today's most widespread diseases have one common denominator: long-term vitamin deficiencies. The time had come to shape this new understanding as the broad scientific concept of Cellular Medicine, which has become the foundation of a new era of health care.

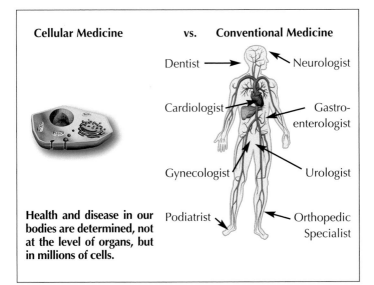

**Cellular Medicine**     vs.     **Conventional Medicine**

Dentist — Neurologist

Cardiologist — Gastroenterologist

Gynecologist — Urologist

Podiatrist — Orthopedic Specialist

**Health and disease in our bodies are determined, not at the level of organs, but in millions of cells.**

253

There are three main elements of Cellular Medicine that set this new health concept fundamentally apart from conventional medicine:

## 1. Cells vs. Organs:

Health and disease are not determined at the level of organs, but at the level of millions of cells composing these organs. The long-term dietary deficiency of vitamins and other biocatalysts for cellular metabolism are the most frequent cause of cellular malfunction and disease.

## 2. Cause vs. Symptoms:

Most pharmaceutical drugs are merely symptom oriented. Accordingly, pharmaceutical-dependent conventional medicine has limited options for prevention, root cause treatment or elimination of diseases. In sharp contrast, the target of Cellular Medicine is to correct the impaired metabolism of cells, thereby allowing effective prevention, treatment and, eventually, elimination of the disease.

## 3. Patient Control vs. Dependency:

Cellular Medicine not only allows millions of patients to understand the causes of diseases, but also gives them the means to correct these causes in the form of specific vitamins and essential nutrients. Conventional medicine frequently relies on Latin language to make it impossible for the patient to understand the cause of disease and creates dependencies on the therapeutic options offered by drug companies. In contrast, Cellular Medicine educates the patient about the basic functions of the body, the primary causes of diseases and the basic therapeutic options for prevention and correction. Thus, Cellular Medicine becomes the tool for millions of patients to liberate themselves from the deadlock of pharmaceutical medicine.

Cellular Medicine has become the scientific basis for health liberation not only for millions of patients, but also for the implementation of effective and affordable public health measures in many nations. In fact, Cellular Medicine has become synonymous with the worldwide transformation of profit-oriented medicine toward patient-oriented health care.

After the discovery of the nature of cardiovascular disease, the next milestone of Cellular Medicine was to identify the natural means to control cancer. Once again, our detailed understanding of cellular function paves the way so that the diagnosis "cancer" is no longer a death verdict for patients. That discovery, too, is being heavily fought because it inevitably destroys one of the most lucrative pharmaceutical markets — toxic cancer drugs (chemotherapy) and the drugs subsequently prescribed to ameliorate the inevitable health damage done by them.

The details of this discovery in cellular cancer research go beyond the scope of this book. They are documented in detail in my book *Cancer* and on our research website at www.dr-rath-research.org. These and other advances in Cellular Medicine are being investigated at our Cellular Medicine Research Institute in California.

Based on the breakthrough discoveries described in this book, we have developed natural health programs, which today are available around the world. At the same time, this medical breakthrough is featured on the Internet. Today, the website www.drrath.com has become the leading resource on the Internet for natural health information.

Of course, a breakthrough of this magnitude triggered massive reactions on the part the pharmaceutical industry, which had to defend its trillion dollar stake. These reactions can be summarized as "fight it" and "use it." The principle reaction of the pharmaceutical industry was to categorically fight this breakthrough in natural health by seeking to impose "protectionist laws," not only in the U.S., but worldwide. Since this would take several years to accomplish, some pharmaceutical companies decided — in the meantime — to take economic advantage of this breakthrough. This criminal conspiracy for the price-fixing of vitamin raw materials is known today as the "Vitamin Cartel."

## Milestone 8: Vitamin Cartel

By the turn of the century, the world's largest pharmaceutical and nutritional companies, including Hofmann-La Roche, BASF, Rhône-Poulenc, Archer Daniels Midland (ADM), Takeda and other multinational corporations, had admitted to forming a so-called "vitamin cartel" to conduct criminal price-fixing for vitamin raw materials. Hundreds of millions of people worldwide were defrauded for almost a decade and had to pay artificially high prices for vitamins and certain other essential nutrients. The U.S. Justice Department declared that this vitamin cartel was the largest cartel ever discovered and named it an "economic conspiracy." Hoffman-La Roche, BASF and the other cartel members agreed to pay more than one billion dollars in fines in the U.S. for committing these crimes.

While the audacity of these criminal practices and the magnitude of this consumer fraud made headlines around the world, no one asked the decisive question: Who or what triggered the formation of this global cartel? Coordinated criminal activities of this nature just don't appear out of nowhere. They are the result of corporate greed, and the direct consequence of events that promised financial benefits for the criminal conspirators that far outweighed any risk of getting caught.

The background of this illegal vitamin cartel is the scientific breakthrough documented in this book in relation to vitamins and the prevention of cardiovascular disease. Already at the beginning of 1990, I had informed Hofmann-La Roche about these discoveries. On June 2, 1990, I sent a summary of the discovery that heart attacks and strokes are — like scurvy — the result of vitamin C deficiency to Professor Jürgen Drews, head of Hofmann-La Roche Research Worldwide and a member of its executive board.

Hofmann-La Roche is the world's leading manufacturer of vitamin C raw material. Hofmann-La Roche executives realized immediately that my discovery would boost their international demand for vitamin C and create a multi-billion dollar market for it and other vitamins. In order to get further information from me, the executives of Hofmann-La Roche signed a confidentiality agreement and invited me to represent the new understanding of heart disease at their global headquarters in Basel, Switzerland. However, Hofmann-La Roche decided *not* to promote this medical breakthrough, despite the fact that they acknowledged it as such. The reasons they gave to me in writing were that Hofmann-La Roche did not want to finance the dissemination of this understanding of heart disease for all their competitors, and they did not want to compete with other in-house pharmaceutical drug developments, such as cholesterol-lowering drugs.

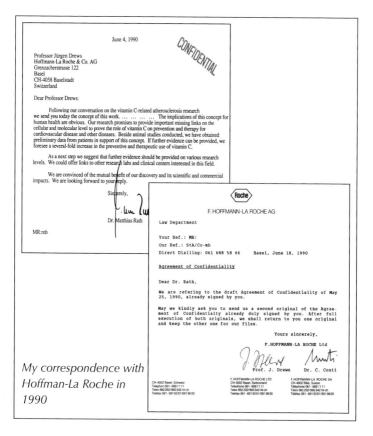

*My correspondence with Hoffman-La Roche in 1990*

Thus, while they refused to promote this medical breakthrough, which could have saved millions of lives, this pharmaceutical company turned around and decided to conspire in the formation of a vitamin cartel in order to take advantage of the breakthrough. Hofmann-La Roche apparently invited BASF, Rhone-Poulenc, Takeda and other manufacturers of vitamin raw materials to engage in criminal price-fixing on a global level. The fraudulent profits these companies made from their criminal practices may have reached hundreds of billions of dollars over the past 10 years. Compared to that, the fines these companies had to pay were insignificant.

Not only should governments have sued these companies for the damage they had done, but above all, consumers worldwide should have filed class action lawsuits against them. These companies have harmed millions of people twice: First, they knowingly refused to promote and disseminate livesaving information about the use of vitamins for the prevention of heart disease, thereby causing millions of heart patients to die unnecessarily over the past 10 years. Second, they caused financial damage to hundreds of millions of people — literally every vitamin consumer on earth.

My correspondence with Hofmann-La Roche executives also proves the statements they and others made that the corporate executives did not know about these criminal activities were lies. The opposite is true: These corporate executives not only knew about these crimes, they were the organizers. The executives responsible for these crimes should be prosecuted and held responsible for their actions.

While that may take time, one benefit is already here today. All these companies have pleaded guilty to criminal activities. Thus, everyone can describe these companies and their executives for what they are — criminals who distinguish themselves from a street robber only by the magnitude of their crimes.

**Milestone 9:  Protecting Natural Health Freedom Against the Pharmaceutical Cartel**

The principal strategy of the globally operating pharmaceutical cartel was the fundamental obstruction of the breakthrough documented in this book. Its primary goal was — and still is — to achieve a global ban on the dissemination of related natural health information and natural therapies.

With the battle to make vitamins prescription items in the U.S. lost, the pharmaceutical industry decided to regroup at the international level. In 1995, they launched a global campaign to outlaw all health information about vitamins and other natural, non-patentable therapies. Toward this end, the pharma-cartel even abuses the international political institutions, such as the European Parliament and the United Nation's "Codex Alimentarius Commission."

The pharma-cartel's Codex plans are a desperate effort by the international pharmaceutical industry to secure its survival as we know it today. If they lose this global battle — similar to the defeat in the U.S. — vitamins will become accepted worldwide as powerful preventive and therapeutic agents that benefit millions of people, and substantially reduce the markets for pharmaceutical drugs.

For almost 10 years now, the pharmaceutical cartel has been coordinating its "Codex" plans in Germany — until recently — the lead export nation of pharmaceutical products. In "closed door meetings," they have been trying to push their plan for a global ban on vitamin therapies through the United Nations with no success. Together with patients and friends of our Health Alliance, we have been able to block these unscrupulous efforts again and again.

In 1996, 1998, 2000, 2001 and 2002, these unscrupulous plans to restrict health freedom worldwide were on the agenda of the Berlin Codex meetings. The main reason why these

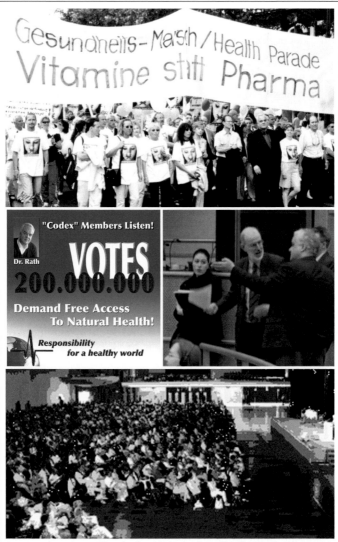

*Images from our "Battle for Vitamin Freedom" (top to bottom): Codex 2000: Rally in Berlin; Codex 2001: 200 million emails for vitamin freedom; EU Parliament 2002: Dr. Rath hands over the petition for vitamin freedom to the vice president of the EU Parliament; Codex 2002: Natural Health Symposium in Berlin.*

plans could not be passed were our protests against them. These protests came in different forms, including rallies, health conferences, Open Letters in newspapers, info-mailings, letters by patients to Codex delegates and many other actions. Particularly effective were petition drives in the form of email campaigns. In 2002, the number of emails sent to Codex members, politicians and governments supporting the Codex plans of the pharma-cartel surpassed 650 million from around the world.

In parallel efforts, the drug companies were also trying to abuse national parliaments, as well as regional institutions. Most recently, they twisted the arm of the European Parliament and its cabinet (European Commission). On the day in March 2002 when the vote on the restriction of natural health for the people of Europe was voted on, so many protest emails arrived at the EU Parliament that the entire email system was shut down — for the first time in its history.

What have we accomplished with these protests? A lot! First, we have prevented the unethical pharma-cartel plans for a global ban on natural therapies from being implemented long ago. Second, we have convinced Codex delegates from South Africa and other countries, primarily from the developing world, that by supporting the pharma-cartel's Codex plans, they are not solving, but actually aggravating the health problems in their countries and increasing the dependency on the pharma-cartel.

Most importantly, we have informed millions of people about these unscrupulous plans. These people, among them scientists, doctors and politicians, were enabled to see behind the deceptive smoke screen of "consumer protection" and "trade standards" drawn up by the pharma-cartel as a pretense for their protectionist laws.

Many times during those years, I gave speeches on behalf of the people of the world. I spoke for millions of people in America, Asia, Africa and Europe. I spoke for the present generation and for generations yet to come. All these millions had one thing in common: the unscrupulous plans of the pharma-cartel directly affected their health and lives, and many of them did not even know about it.

When the history pages about the liberation of human health are one day written, they will be about the years when this liberation was most threatened. I am not asking you where you were all those years. Reading this book may be the first time that you have heard about the unethical plans of the pharma-cartel. But now that you have learned about it, I am asking you: "What are you going to do?"

One thing is clear: Without you speaking out for your very own health interests, the pharmaceutical interest groups may still reverse everything we have accomplished so far. After reading this book, you will no longer be able to say that you did not know.

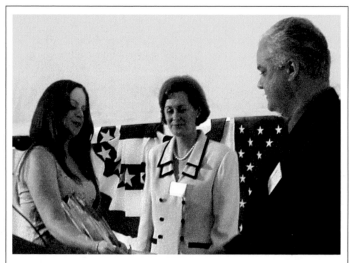

*In May 2001, I received the Bulwark of Liberty Award from the American Association of Preventive Medicine "in recognition of extraordinary efforts to advance nutrition science, to educate the public on the health benefits of nutrients and to end government censorship of health information."*

## Milestone 10: Building a Health Alliance

There is no doubt: The turn from the second to the third millennium coincides with a change in health care worldwide. Millions of people are waking up and realizing that they have become dependent on a deceptive health concept that is little more than an illusion. The fact that it took so long to unmask this fraud is no surprise, either. Those who benefit financially from this deception — the pharmaceutical industry — are doing everything to cover it up. The information in this book has been a key factor in bringing the truth to light. Now that the scientific facts can no longer be suppressed, patients and health professionals are taking advantage of these breakthroughs in natural health. Tens of thousands of people worldwide are already working in our international Health Alliance with the goal of implementing a new health care system —irrespective of where they live.

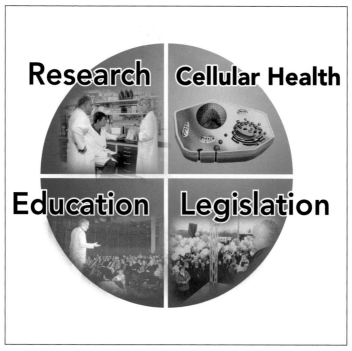

# Why We Need Dr. Rath's Health Alliance

In a world where the health care sector is the monopoly of those who make money from ongoing diseases, you should not expect that health will be offered to you voluntarily. In fact, you have to defend your health against those financial interests, and you have to fight for your right to stay healthy.

If you think this statement is too strong, consider the history of the largest health organization on earth, the World Health Organization (WHO). This world body was founded in 1948 with the purpose of improving health on a global level. Until the early 1960s, the main focus of WHO's efforts to reach this goal was the dissemination of information about the health value of nutrition, including vitamins and other essential nutrients.

It took the pharmaceutical cartel little more than a decade to infiltrate this world body and remodel it into its exact opposite. Consequently, for the last 40 years, WHO has been an instrument of the pharmaceutical industry and its quest to expand its global drug market. Abusing WHO, the pharma-cartel first marginalized nutritional programs and education in this field, and is now even openly fighting them in the form of Codex Alimentarius and other means. Toward the same goal, the pharma-cartel has infiltrated the health care sectors and their decision makers in every country.

These facts demonstrate the need for immediate change. They also indicate that it would be unwise to wait for these established institutions to bring about this change. They cannot do it without reforming themselves.

As a result, I decided to create an alliance of people committed to improving their own health and the health of others in their communities and countries. I gave this organization the name "Dr. Rath's Health Alliance."

# The Goals of Dr. Rath's Health Alliance

There are four main areas of activities for our Alliance:

1. **Improving your own health and the health of others** by taking advantage of the discoveries in Cellular Medicine described in this book.

2. **Promoting research in natural health and Cellular Medicine:** Our Cellular Medicine Research Institute focuses on a continuous effort to document the health benefits of vitamins and other nutrients essential for optimum cellular function.

3. **Promoting health education at the community and national levels:** Since television and other mass media are reluctant to give up their most profitable relationships with the pharmaceutical "business with disease," there is only one other way: — you must help to spread this lifesaving information yourself. We encourage you to turn your living room or another suitable room in your house into a "consulting center" for Cellular Health.

4. **Protecting your health freedom from being compromised on behalf of the pharmaceutical "business with disease":** This area of activity includes our commitment to stop legislation — whether national or international — that takes away our health choices and our freedom to access natural health information.

Most of our Alliance members are patients who have experienced the deadlock of conventional medicine for decades. With the help of vitamin research and our Cellular Medicine formulas, these patients have regained lives worth living. Many thousands of these patients in Europe, America and other continents are living proof that a new health care system has already become reality.

But I am not only inviting patients. Whoever you are and wherever you live, if you want to take responsibility for your own health and help improve the heath of others, I invite you to join us.

# How You Can Learn More About Cellular Health

True health starts with knowledge. If you do not know how your body works and how the cells of your body function properly, you will not be able to stay healthy. Instead, you will remain illiterate about the most important question of your life — your health — and this illiteracy will keep you dependent on those who promote the pharmaceutical "business with disease" at the expense of your health.

There is an easy way to change this. You simply need to learn the basics about Cellular Health and the natural pevention of diseases. By reading this book, you are taking an important first step. But there is much more to learn.

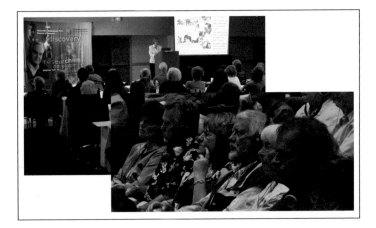

I invite you to attend one of our Cellular Health Education Seminars. They are for people who want to know more — people like you. There, you will learn about the benefits of micronutrients in maintaining health and how you can apply this knowledge to help yourself and others. The seminar also provides information about the most common deadlocks of pharmaceutical-based conventional medicine.

What you learn at the Cellular Health Education Seminar will empower you with the knowledge you need to take control of your health. As a result of this knowledge, you may feel encouraged to take on a new career as a consultant for natural health care.

By participating in our seminars, you can acquire an education certificate as a "Cellular Health Consultant," and show others that you are willing to share your natural health knowledge by directing them to the road of optimum health.

For details, please visit our website at **www.dr-rath-research.org**

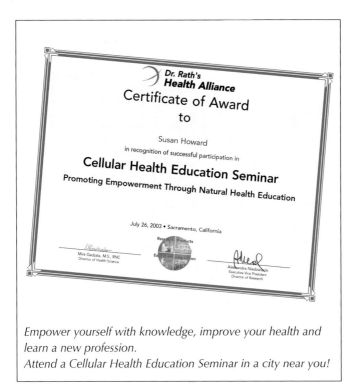

*Empower yourself with knowledge, improve your health and learn a new profession.*
*Attend a Cellular Health Education Seminar in a city near you!*

---

**Comments About Our Cellular Health Education Seminars**

*"Do not let the pharmaceutical industry win!"*

*"We should tell others about Dr. Rath's discoveries and this great seminar."*

*"I learned from this seminar how diseases start and can be prevented."*

---

# What You Can Do Immediately

- Pass this book on to relatives, neighbors, colleagues, friends and your doctor.

- Contact your local newspapers, radio and TV stations in order to help spread this information through the media.

- Sign the "Petition for Vitamin Freedom" (see Chapter 12), and urge others to support it with their signatures.

- Contact your city council and other political representatives. Attach a short letter in support of these documents and add your own comments.

This new era of human health will be based on health information, education and health empowerment of the public at large. Patients and laypeople will become natural health consultants, and consulting centers for Cellular Medicine will be created. I encourage you to become an architect of this new health care system.

# Principles of a New Health Care System

1. **Health is understandable for everyone.** The basic concepts of human health and disease can be understood by *everyone*. The fact that millions of body cells regularly need vitamins and other bioenergy carriers can even be grasped by children.

2. **Health is doable for everyone.** Cellular Medicine and the daily intake of vitamins and other bioenergy carriers allow *everyone* to maintain and restore basic physical health.

3. **Health is safe for everyone.** Nature itself provides us with vitamins and other powerful preventive and therapeutic substances to combat human diseases. They are safe for everyone and without side effects.

4. **Health is affordable for everyone.** Effective health measures to prevent the most common human diseases can be offered in any country of the world at a fraction of today's drug costs. Implementation of Cellular Medicine as a health measure immediately liberates trillions of dollars in private and public funds.

5. **Health is a human right.** Having access to optimum health is a basic human right. No pharmaceutical company or government has the right to limit the spread of information about the health benefits of vitamins and other natural therapies. Every country in the world should amend its constitution to guarantee access to optimum health to its citizens.

6. **Effective health care focuses on prevention.** Future medical research and health care will focus on the prevention and eradication of diseases rather than on therapies that merely relieve the symptoms of diseases.

7. **Effective health care focuses on primary health care.** Community-based primary health care is the key to effective and affordable health care in any country of the world. Health consultants and health centers in every community will replace the ineffective and expensive focus on high-tech medicine.

8. **Medical research has to be under public control.** Public funds for medical research should primarily be used to develop treatments that *prevent* and *eradicate* diseases, rather than ones that merely relieve symptoms and create dependencies.

# Notes

# 12

Nutrition

Saturday May 4, 20

# Documentation

- The Lecture at Stanford Medical School
- The Scurvy-Heart Disease Connection
- "Health for All by the Year 2020"
- "The Hague Constitution"
- Petition for Vitamin Freedom
- About the Author
- Clinical Study: Natural Reversal of Heart Disease
- References

# The Lecture at Stanford Medical School

On May 4, 2002, I was privileged to give the following lecture at a symposium on nutrition at Stanford Medical School in Palo Alto, California.

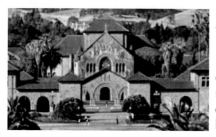

For more than a century, this medical institution has gracefully served the interests of the pharmaceutical cartel by promoting its multi-billion dollar business with heart disease.

For more than a decade, the pharmaceutical cartel has vigorously fought my discovery of the scurvy-heart disease connection, realizing that it threatens the very basis of this business. In that fight, they have also abused many medical opinion leaders.

Now, the growing acceptance of the scurvy-heart disease connection can no longer be ignored. My lecture at Stanford University was a historic event because it broke the stranglehold of the pharmaceutical cartel on established medical institutions. The doctors who organized the event deserve some credit for opening these closely guarded gates of medicine.

Twenty minutes of my lecture felt like an earthquake to the house of cards that is pharmaceutical cardiology. Cellular Medicine has now opened the doors for new generations of doctors and cardiologists, enabling them to save millions of lives.

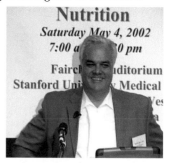

*Delivering my lecture at Stanford University*

272

# The Scurvy-Heart Disease Connection:
## Solution to the Puzzle of Cardiovascular Disease

"I would like to congratulate Stanford University for addressing the need for preventive and natural answers to the number one cause of death in the industrialized world. I will present to you the facts that atherosclerosis, heart attacks and strokes are not diseases, but the direct result of long-term vitamin deficiency. And, therefore, they can be prevented by natural means, without pharmaceutical drugs or surgical intervention.

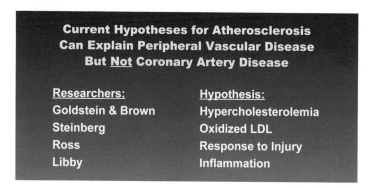

Heart disease is an early form of the sailor's disease scurvy. In my presentation, I can only focus on the most compelling evidence. For more details, I encourage you to visit our research website www.dr-rath-research.org.

All existing hypotheses of atherogenesis have one problem in common — they defy human logic. If high cholesterol levels, oxidized LDL or bacteria damage the vascular wall, atherosclerotic plaques would occur along the entire vascular pipeline. Inevitably, peripheral vascular disease would be the primary manifestation of cardiovascular disease. This is clearly not the case.

It doesn't require a degree from Stanford or any other medical school — any layperson can solve the 'Football Field Riddle.'

273

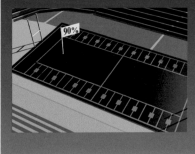

## The "Football Field Riddle"

The total surface area of the blood vessel system in a person is comparable to the size of a football field.

But in 90% of the cases, it clogs in the same small spot — the size of the marker for the "extra point" kick.

The arteries, veins and capillaries in our bodies compose a pipeline that is 60,000 miles long and covers the area of a football field. But this pipeline fails in 90% of the cases at one specific spot: the coronary arteries, which are the length of only one billionth of the total vascular pipeline. If high cholesterol — or any other risk factor circulating in the bloodstream — could cause damage to this pipeline, it would clog everywhere, not just at one spot. Obviously, elevated cholesterol cannot be the primary cause of coronary artery disease.

The solution to the puzzle of cardiovascular disease, therefore, must lie in the explanation of coronary artery plaques as the predominant manifestation of cardiovascular disease. To solve this puzzle, we need to refocus our attention away from the bloodstream and its constituents to the one and only relevant target: the stability of the vascular wall.

The following picture shows the connection between cardiovascular disease and the sailor's disease scurvy. Unlike animals, the human body cannot synthesize vitamin C. Ascorbate deficiency results in two distinct morphological changes in the vascular wall: impaired vascular stability due to decreased collagen synthesis and loss of the endothelial barrier function.

# The "Scurvy-Heart Disease Connection"

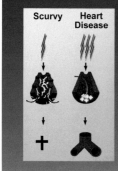

Scurvy     Heart
           Disease

Cardiovascular disease is an early form of the sailor's disease scurvy. In both cases, lack of vitamin C in the vascular cells is the underlying problem.

In scurvy, a complete depletion of ascorbate in the body dissolves the structure of the blood vessel wall causing leaks, blood loss, and eventually death.

In cardiovascular disease, ascorbate deficiency gradually develops over decades, allowing time for vascular repair mechanisms (plaque formation).

The sailors of earlier centuries died within a few months from hemorrhagic blood loss due to a lack of endogenous ascorbate synthesis combined with a vitamin-deficient diet. When the Indians gave those sailors tea from tree barks and other vitamin-rich nutrition, blood loss was stopped and the vascular wall healed naturally. Thus, the damage was repaired!

Today, we all get *some* vitamin C in the diet, and open scurvy is rare. But it is not enough, and almost everyone suffers from chronic vitamin deficiency. Over decades, microscopic lesions develop along the vascular wall, especially in areas of high mechanical stress, such as the coronary arteries (pumping heart).

Just as in the sailor's disease scurvy, vitamin C induces the natural repair of the blood vessel wall in cardiovascular disease, leading to a halt in the progression and even to the natural regression of vascular lesions.

In contrast to current models of atherogenesis, the 'Scurvy-Heart Disease Connection' answers all the key questions in cardiology today.

**1. Why do we get infarctions of the heart and not of the nose or ears?**

The answer can be reduced to two factors: structural impairment of the vascular wall due to vitamin deficiency combined

275

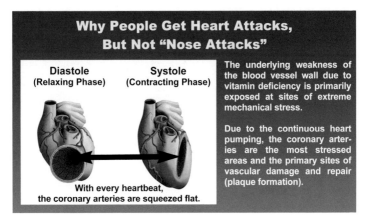

with the mechanical stress from pulsatile blood flow in the coronary arteries. It is at this unique spot where the underlying structural impairment is exposed first.

## 2. Why do we get arteriosclerosis, but not venosclerosis?

The hypothesis that cholesterol, bacterial infections, chlamydia and other blood risk factors cause plaques would inevitably also lead to clogging of veins and lead to *veno*sclerosis. This is clearly not the case. The scurvy-heart disease connection provides the only logical answer to this question.

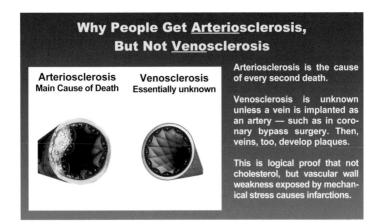

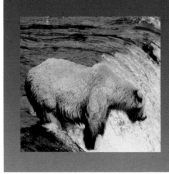

## Why Animals Don't Get Heart Attacks

With the rarest of exceptions, animals don't develop arteriosclerosis.

Prominent examples are bears. They have average blood cholesterol levels of about 600 mg/dl. They don't get heart attacks because they produce their own vitamin C, which stabilizes their artery walls.

### 3. Why don't animals get heart attacks, but people do?

Why are bears and other hibernators with cholesterol levels of 600 mg/dl not extinct from an epidemic of heart attacks? The answer: Animals produce their own vitamin C in amounts between one gram and 20 grams (six teaspoons) each day, compared to the human body weight. These amounts of ascorbate are obviously sufficient to optimize the stability of their vascular walls — without any necessity for statins and other cholesterol lowering drugs.

### 4. Why are all important risk factors for cardiovascular disease closely connected to ascorbate deficiency?

All risk factors for cardiovascular disease known today, including:

• carbohydrate metabolism — such as diabetes
• lipid metabolism — high cholesterol and other hyperlipidemias
• amino acid metabolism — such as homocysteinuria

are closely connected to deficiencies in vitamin C and other micronutrients essential for vascular cell metabolism. The common denominator of these metabolic disorders is to provide compensatory stability for the vitamin-deficient vascular wall. This is also the reason why ascorbate deficiency increases fibrinogen and thromboxane levels while decreasing endothelial-derived relaxing factors (NO) and prostacyclin.

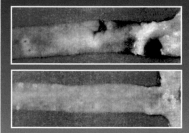

## The "Guinea Pig Proof"

Like humans, guinea pigs cannot produce their own vitamin C.

With low vitamin C in their diets, these animals develop atherosclerotic plaques structurally identical to human atherosclerosis.

When fed a daily amount of vitamin C equivalent to 5 grams, the arteries were protected and did not show any plaques.

Let's consider the key evidence for the scurvy-heart disease connection. The guinea pig, like man, cannot synthesize ascorbate endogenously. In our research published in the *Proceedings of the National Academy of Sciences*, we demonstrated that when guinea pigs were fed vitamin C only at the level of the human RDA, they developed atherosclerosis. These vascular lesions were histologically indistinguishable from human atherosclerotic plaques. In contrast, animals that received about one teaspoon of vitamin C per day had clean arteries.

These experiments were confirmed by Dr. Maeda and her colleagues in an ascorbate 'knock-out' animal model. The first manifestation in these animals was the deterioration of the vascular wall, which resembled early atherosclerosis in humans.

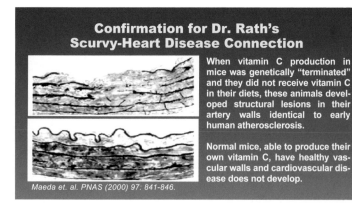

## Confirmation for Dr. Rath's Scurvy-Heart Disease Connection

When vitamin C production in mice was genetically "terminated" and they did not receive vitamin C in their diets, these animals developed structural lesions in their artery walls identical to early human atherosclerosis.

Normal mice, able to produce their own vitamin C, have healthy vascular walls and cardiovascular disease does not develop.

*Maeda et. al. PNAS (2000) 97: 841-846.*

## Clinical Proof From
## Coronary Heart Disease Patients

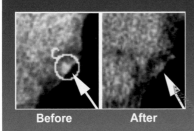

**Before**      **After**

For the first time in medicine, the natural reversal of coronary heart disease was documented by X-ray pictures (Ultrafast Computed Tomography).

In this patient, the coronary artery plaques had entirely disappeared after one year of following my cellular nutrient program.

We confirmed these results in a clinical study in patients with existing coronary artery deposits measured by Ultrafast Computed Tomography. Following a defined vitamin program, the progression of calcification significantly decreased and, in some cases, the disappearance of lesions was documented, as you can see in the X-ray CT pictures. (The publication of this clinical study is documented at the end of this book.)

The scurvy-heart disease connection means a paradigm shift in medicine from targeting symptoms to the only relevant preventive and therapeutic target: the stability of the vascular wall. With the discovery of the scurvy-heart disease connection, the 'universe of heart disease' has ceased to be a 'plate' and has become a 'globe.'

## The Scurvy-Heart Disease Connection
## Turns the "Universe of Heart Disease"
## From a Plate Into a Globe

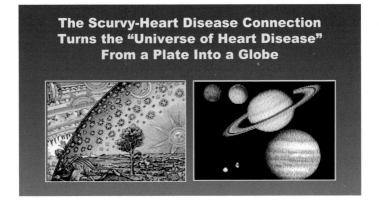

Now that we have identified the true nature of cardiovascular disease, its eradication is only a question of time. Ten years from now, the headlines of leading newspapers may read:

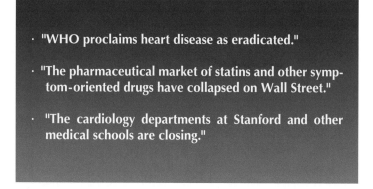

· "WHO proclaims heart disease as eradicated."

· "The pharmaceutical market of statins and other symptom-oriented drugs have collapsed on Wall Street."

· "The cardiology departments at Stanford and other medical schools are closing."

On behalf of millions of patients with heart disease, I call upon Stanford University and other medical institutions to accept their responsibility and join us in the eradication of cardiovascular disease." *(End of lecture)*

## Reactions to My Lecture

**Question by John Cook, Ph.D., M.D., Professor of Cardiology and organizer of this conference at Stanford Medical School:** Dr. Rath, you mentioned something that is very interesting. In fact, I think it is the $64,000 question: Why does one develop atherosclerosis? Why is there a special heterogeneity (variation) in atherosclerosis? I think that's an important point. I feel it is because of differences in the systems, in that the veins and arteries are quite different. Certainly, they are subjected to different hemodynamic (blood flow) forces, and actually they are derived from different tissues, the veins, capillaries and so forth, and my own feeling is that would explain the special heterogeneity, as well as the hemodynamic forces.

**Dr. Rath:** Well, if you take a coronary bypass operation, for example, a *vein* is taken from the leg and that blood vessel is implanted as a coronary *artery* on top of the heart. From that moment on, this vein is subjected to pulsatile (pumping) blood flow. The former vein is now functioning as an artery, and it develops atherosclerotic plaques that eventually can clog this blood vessel.

**Comment by another professor of cardiology:** But we also have studies that show little or no effect of vitamins on cardio-vascular disease.

**Dr. Rath:** Who is "we"? If you go to the medical libraries on the Internet, you will find over 10,000 studies documenting the health benefits of vitamins. Moreover, the greatest study ever conducted on Planet Earth has revealed that in billions of animals, cardiovascular disease is essentially unknown because they produce their own vitamin C.

The question is how long are you willing to ignore the facts and risk that millions of people will continue to die from a disease that could be long gone? So, who is "we"?

"My dear Kepler, what do you say of the leading philosophers here to whom I have offered a thousand times of my own accord to show my studies, but who, with the lazy obstinacy of a serpent who has eaten his fill, have never consented to look at the planets, or moon, or telescope? Verily, just as serpents close their eyes, so do men close their eyes to the light of truth."

Galileo Galilei in a letter to Johannes Kepler, 1630

# Eradicating Heart Disease Is Possible!

### Rath-Pauling Call to Eradicate Heart Disease

On July 2, 1992, for the first time ever, the possibility of eradicating heart disease from mankind was publicly announced. In his last public appeal, the two-time Nobel Laureate Linus Pauling supported my scientific breakthrough in heart disease research.

Only weeks later, the pharmaceutical cartel launched its legislative efforts via the FDA (Food and Drug Administration) to suppress this breakthrough and to make vitamins prescription drugs. In the "battle for vitamin freeedom" of 1992-1994, the people in the U.S. prevented these unscrupulous plans and defended their health rights.

*A Call for an International Effort to Abolish Heart Disease*

*Heart disease, stroke, and other forms of cardiovascular disease now kill millions of people every year and cause millions more to be disabled. There now exists the opportunity to reduce greatly this toll of death and disability by the optimum dietary supplementation with vitamins and other essential nutrients.*

*THE GOAL OF ELIMINATING HEART DISEASE AS THE MAJOR CAUSE OF DEATH AND DISABILITY IS NOW IN SIGHT!*

*Matthias Rath and Linus Pauling*

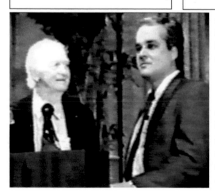

**Above:** *Two handwritten pages from the last public appeal of the two-time Nobel Laureate before his death in 1994.*

**Left:** *Dr. Pauling and myself at the historic press conference in San Francisco, July 2, 1992, announcing "A Call for an International Effort to Abolish Heart Disease."*

282

# CALL FOR AN INTERNATIONAL EFFORT
# TO ABOLISH HEART DISEASE

Heart disease, stroke and other forms of cardiovascular disease now kill millions of people every year and cause millions more to be disabled. There now exists the opportunity to reduce greatly this toll of death and disability by the optimum dietary supplementation with vitamins and other essential nutrients.

During recent years, we and our associates have made two remarkable discoveries. One is that the primary cause of heart disease is the insufficient intake of ascorbate (vitamin C), an insufficiency from which nearly every person on earth suffers. Ascorbate deficiency leads to weakness of the walls of the arteries and the initiation of the atherosclerotic process, particularly in stressed regions. We conclude that cholesterol and other blood risk factors increase the risk for heart disease only if the wall of the artery is weakened by ascorbate deficiency.

The other discovery is that the main cholesterol-transporting particle forming atherosclerotic plaques is not LDL (low-density lipoprotein) but a related lipoprotein, lipoprotein (a). Moreover, certain essential nutrients, especially the amino acid L-lysine, can block the deposition of this lipoprotein and may even reduce existing plaques. We have concluded that the optimum supplementation of ascorbate and some other nutrients could largely prevent heart disease and stroke and be effective in treating existing disease. Published clinical and epidemiological data support this conclusion.

The goal is now in sight: the abolition of heart disease as the cause of disability and mortality for the present generation and future generations of human beings.

### WITH MILLIONS OF LIVES EACH YEAR AT STAKE,
### NO TIME SHOULD BE LOST!

- We call upon our colleagues in science and medicine to join in a vigorous international effort, on the levels of both basic research and clinical studies, to investigate the value of vitamin C and other nutrients in controlling heart disease.
- We call upon national and international health authorities and other health institutions to support this effort with political and financial measures.
- We call upon every human being to encourage local medical institutions and physicians to take an active part in this process.

### THE GOAL OF ELIMINATING HEART DISEASE AS THE MAJOR
### CAUSE OF DEATH AND DISABILITY IS NOW IN SIGHT!

*Matthias Rath and Linus Pauling*
San Francisco, California, July 1992

283

## "Health for All by the Year 2020" Is Possible!

### Dr. Rath's Call to Political Leaders, World Summit 2002

After 10 years of a series of Cellular Medicine breakthroughs, it is clear that Cellular Medicine can help control today's most common diseases. At the World Summit in Johannesburg in August 2002, I called upon the world community to take advantage of these breakthroughs.

# Health For All

The Dr. Rath Health Foundation is dedicated to promoting natural health information and to protecting the right to natural health against the global interests of the pharmaceutical industry.

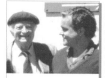

Dr. Matthias Rath, M.D., is the world renowned scientist and physician who led the scientific breakthrough towards *natural* prevention and treatment of cardiovascular disease and more recently cancer. His discoveries have already saved many lives around the world.

*The late two-time Nobel Laureate Dr. Linus Pauling, who considered Dr. Rath as his successor stated: "Dr. Raths discoveries rank among the most important discoveries in medicine."*

Dr. Rath leads an internationally recognized independent research institute dedicated to eliminate today's most common diseases with effective, natural and affordable therapies.

Dr. Rath is member of the American Heart Association (AHA), the New York Academy of Sciences and other international organizations.

In 2001 he has been awarded the "Bulwark of Liberty Award" from the American Association of Preventive Medicine for his courage to stand up against the plans of the pharmaceutical industry to ban natural health information world-wide by abusing the United Nation's "Codex Alimentarius Commission".

1. **Health is a basic human right.** Every person is entitled to make use of this right without any restriction. Public institutions and private organizations are to be held accountable for providing life-saving health information to the people of the world. The obstruction of the right to essential health information for everyone constitutes a crime against humanity.

2. **Today, health is not available to every human being for good reasons.** They include social injustice, military conflicts and others. Another significant reason is the fact that the most profitable industry on earth, the pharmaceutical industry, is an investment industry based upon the existence and continuation of diseases - despite declarations to the contrary. Low-cost prevention, treatment and elimination of diseases threaten this multi-trillion dollar "business with disease".

3. **Most efforts to improve health on a global scale have failed thus far.** The World Health Organization's effort "Health for All by the Year 2000" could not reach its goals because it did not distinctly separate itself from the global "business with disease." It focused instead on administrative health care changes, rather than taking advantage of global advances in medicine.

4. **Advances in the field of natural medicine have been made over recent years** that will reduce the incidence of common diseases in the industrialized countries as well as in the developing world, to a fraction of their current frequency. The primary cause of the world's most common health conditions is a chronic deficiency of micronutrients, essential for optimum cellular energy metabolism as well as optimum connective tissue stability.

5. **In the industrialized world,** the leading causes of death are heart attacks, cancer, strokes, diabetes and high blood pressure. Using the available knowledge in nutritional

**For more information, vis**

These breakthroughs can also be applied to fight major health problems in the developing world, including AIDS and other infectious diseases. The Dr. Rath Health Foundation promotes effective and affordable natural health information with the goal of building a new global health care system to provide "health for all by the year 2020."

# By The Year 2020

research and cellular medicine, these health conditions can be significantly reduced and hundreds of millions of lives can be saved.

6. **In the developing world,** two billion people suffer from deficiencies in micronutrients, according to United Nations Organizations. Avitaminosis is a leading cause of disease resulting in blindness in millions and promoting infectious diseases in hundreds of millions by compromising cellular defense mechanisms in their bodies. Taking advantage of the knowledge in nutritional medicine already available today, billions of lives can be saved in the developing world.

7. **The eradication of today's most common health problems is dependent on one factor only: how fast the information about this breakthrough in natural health can be spread.** While the scientific knowledge to combat these diseases effectively is available and the essential nutrients to prevent these health conditions, can be produced at low costs, in any quantity, anywhere in the world, the dissemination of this live-saving information to the people of the world is being obstructed.

8. **The Pharmceutical industry tries to protect its global drug market by outlawing natural remedies.** Effective, non-patentable and affordable natural health approaches threaten the very existence of the pharmaceutical industry. The multi-trillion dollar global pharmaceutical market is dependent on synthetic drugs that allow an excessively high return on investment based on the patentability of those drugs. To secure the continued existence of the pharmaceutical industry as the most profitable industry on earth, large corporations embarked on a global battle to outlaw the dissemination of natural health information. To that effect the pharmaceutical industry abuses the United Nations "Codex Alimentarius Commission" and other national and international bodies.

9. **The people of the world face one of the largest challenges in human history.** The right to health and life for billions of people is being threatened by the profit interests of a few shareholders. The goals of these two interest groups are incompatible by their very nature. Similarly, in the battle to save human lives against the profits from patented drugs, every government, every public and private institution has to take a decision on which side they stand. And they will be held accountable by history.

10. **The goal "Health for All by the Year 2020" is in sight.** What is needed immediately is a worldwide effort to promote the dissemination of natural health benefits in every country.

I call upon

• **The United Nations Organizations** and other international organizations to promote natural health policies by all means available;

• **Politicians** in every country to implement natural health as an integral part of national health policies;

• **Health professionals** to utilize natural health approaches to improve the health of your patients.

**I call upon every man and woman to spread this live-saving information in order to protect your life and that of millions of others.**

Johannesburg,
August 2002
Matthias Rath, M.D.

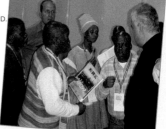

**ww.dr-rath-health-foundation.org**

285

# Health and Peace — Not Disease and War!

*Text from my worldwide Open Letter Series in February/March* 2003: Ten years ago, the late Linus Pauling said to me: "Your discoveries are so important for millions of people that they threaten entire industries. One day there may even be wars just to prevent this breakthrough from being widely accepted. This is the time when you need to stand up!" That time is now!

*Text from my Open Letter published first on February 28, 2003 in the New York Times:*

Today, millions of people worldwide are waking up to the fact that the pharmaceutical industry is an investment industry based on the continuation of diseases. The survival of the pharmaceutical investment industry is threatened by four main factors:

**1** Unsolvable <u>business</u> conflicts. The nature of the pharmaceutical investment industry is the "business with disease." Its basis is the patentability of new synthetic drugs that merely target symptoms, but do not eliminate the root cause of diseases. The continued existence of diseases and their expansion is a precondition for further growth of this industry. Prevention and eradication of diseases undermine the economic basis of this business.

**2** Unsolvable <u>legal</u> conflicts. A wave of patient litigation against the deadly side effects of pharmaceutical drugs threatens to cripple this industry. An end to this litigation is not in sight, since drug side effects are the fourth leading cause of death in the industrialized world. Side effects of pharmaceutical drugs kill more Americans every year than WWII and the Vietnam War combined.

**3** Unsolvable <u>ethical</u> conflicts. The pharmaceutical industry faces an intrinsic conflict between maintaining profits from patent fees and meeting the health needs of people. In developing countries, the profitability of drugs has been a major factor contributing to the spread of AIDS and other epidemics.

**4** Unsolvable <u>scientific</u> conflicts. Advances in vitamin research, Cellular Medicine and natural health allow the control of today's most common diseases. These safe, effective and affordable natural therapies focus on the prevention and eradication of diseases, not only the alleviation of symptoms. This fact and the low profitability of these non-patentable natural approaches threaten the economic base of the pharmaceutical investment business.

**The war against Iraq is not primarily about fighting "terrorism" or conquering oil fields. It is part of a long-term strategy of the pharmaceutical/petrochemical investment groups to create the psychological state of fear to maintain global control.**

286

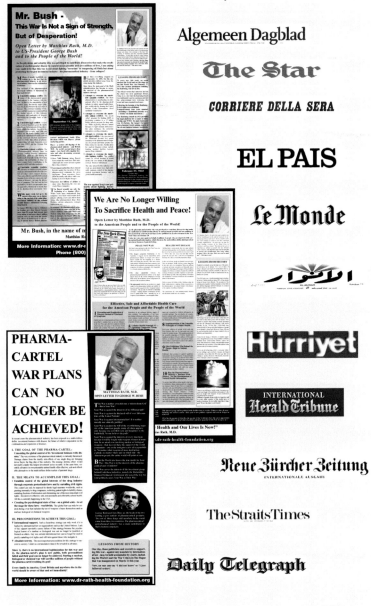

# Blueprint for a Healthy World

On Sunday, March 23, 2003, on the eve of the 2003 Academy Awards ("the Oscars") ceremony in Los Angeles, I published another "Call to Action" in the *Los Angeles Times*, the largest newspaper in that city. The people of Los Angeles and celebrities from around the world took this message home.

This public information exposed to a global audience that the precondition for the eradication of today's most common health problems is the termination of the investment "business with disease" organized around the Rockefeller investment group. For almost a century, these special interest groups have strategically built the most profitable investment industry on earth — at the expense of the health and lives of millions. To achieve their goals, they have abused all sectors of society, including medicine, the media, governments and even the largest political bodies on earth, such as the World Health Organization (WHO).

## Los Angeles Times

March 23, 2003

The war against Iraq has just started and there is already a winner: the people of the World. Over the past weeks, we have informed the people in America and the rest of the World about the background of this war and its main corporate benefactor - the pharmaceutical industry.

This information was first published in the *New York Times*, in the city where political leaders had congregated at the United Nations over the recent months like rarely before in history. International tension and the escalation to war created a climate where the information about the pharmaceutical industry as the main benefactor of the 'war against terrorism' spread like a bush fire.

The global spread of this information was also an important reason why small countries in the Security Council - unexpectedly - resisted the pressure by the United States and British administrations, denying them any mandate and any support by international law for their war.

Now, the war led by the Bush and Blair administrations can no longer reach its primary political and economic goal - that is to impose the monopoly of the multi-trillion dollar pharmaceutical investment "business with disease" on the people of this planet for generations to come.

As the scientist whose discoveries enable us to control today's most common diseases by natural means and having unmasked the corporate benefactors behind the current war, I consider it my responsibility to issue a call to the people and the political leaders of the World to immediately start building a 'World without Disease'!

## Los Angeles Times, March 23, 2003

# Health for All by the Year 2020

Mankind now has an unique opportunity to liberate itself from today's most common diseases.

### A BREATH-TAKING PERSPECTIVE

- **Cardiovascular disease** has been identified as the result of a structural impairment of the blood vessel wall similar to the sailor's disease scurvy. Optimum supply of vitamin C and other micronutrients that stimulate the production of collagen - the vascular reinforcement molecules - is an effective, safe and affordable way to prevent heart attacks and strokes. Thus, the number one cause of death in the industrialized world today can largely be eradicated in this and future generations.

  Global implementation of this scientific knowledge will save millions of lives, billions in health care dollars and eliminate the trillion-dollar pharmaceutical business with cardiovascular disease.

- **High blood pressure, heart failure, irregular heart beat, and diabetic circulatory problems** are primarily the result of long-term micronutrient deficiencies impairing the function of millions of cells that compose the heart muscle and the blood vessel walls.

  Global implementation of this scientific breakthrough will save millions of lives, billions in health care dollars and eliminate the trillion dollar pharmaceutical business with these diseases.

- **Cancer**, the second most frequent cause of death in the industrialized world is no longer a death verdict. All cancer cells spread by using the same mechanism. They produce massive amounts of collagen-digesting enzymes capable of paving their way through the human body during cancer spread.

  Effective, safe and affordable micronutrients such as the amino acid lysine, vitamin C and other specific nutrients block these enzymes and thereby impede cancer disease without any side effects.

  Global implementation of this scientific breakthrough will save millions of lives, billions in health care dollars and eliminate the trillion dollar pharmaceutical business with cancer.

- **Infectious diseases, AIDS and other epidemics** are the leading cause of death in the developing world. B-vitamins and other essential nutrients regulate the production of white blood cells and optimize immune system function in the fight against tuberculosis and other epidemics. Moreover, vitamin C alone has been shown to reduce the multiplication of the AIDS virus to less than 1% of its normal rate. This simple vitamin is more effective than any combination of expensive pharmaceutical drugs.

  Global implementation of this scientific breakthrough will save millions of lives, billions in health care dollars and eliminate the trillion dollar pharmaceutical business with AIDS and other infectious diseases.

In summary, today's most common diseases can now be largely eradicated by natural therapies, thereby improving human health globally and terminating the pharmaceutical investment business with disease.

### WHY THIS DID NOT HAPPEN EARLIER

At the beginning of the 21st century mankind wakes up to a nightmare. A hundred years ago the Rockefeller Group, already controlling the global oil business at that time, defined another global investment market: the human body and the diseases it hosts.

The return on their investment became dependent on the patentability of drugs and the respective patent royalties. Under the umbrella of 'philanthropy' and 'benefactors to mankind' the greatest deception in the history of mankind was strategically developed.

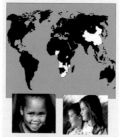

*Every country that focuses its health care system on effective, natural, non-patentable health approaches is an important step towards a healthier and more peaceful world.*

*You can follow the liberation of mankind from the yoke of the pharmaceutical 'investment business with disease' on the Website of our Foundation.*

Millions of patients were promised a 'cure' for their health problems, but the vast majority of the 'remedies' sold had no proven efficacy, at best they covered symptoms. By triggering an epidemic of new diseases from drug side-effects, these deceptive products constantly expanded the 'disease market'.

A strategic precondition for this new market was the elimination of 'competition' from effective natural therapies. The basic knowledge about the essential nutrients required for optimum cellular metabolism was systematically eliminated from medical schools, the textbooks of medicine and from the minds of generations of doctors.

Over several decades the pharmaceutical business with disease became the largest investment industry on planet earth. The huge profits were used to gain influence in all areas of society, including science, medicine, media and politics. Even the largest international bodies did not resist its influence.

### WE NEED A NEW WORLD HEALTH ORGANIZATION

The World Health Organization was founded more than 50 years ago to promote health on a global level. A first focus was to improve health through nutrition, including micronutrients. Within two decades the influence of the pharmaceutical cartel had shifted this focus. By abusing the WHO and other UN organizations (e.g. 'Codex Alimentarius') this industry is trying to impose global protection laws to protect and promote the pharmaceutical investment business with patented drugs from being eliminated by mostly superior, but non-patentable natural therapies.

As the direct result of this silent 'take over' of control of global health care by the pharmaceutical industry during the past century, hundreds of millions of people have died from diseases that could have vanished long ago - if not for the multi-trillion-dollar pharmaceutical investment 'business with disease'. Today, more than two billion people suffer from micronutrient deficiencies in the developing world alone. Thus, all of us must now work towards building a new world health organization that liberates us from today's most common diseases.

### WE NEED A NEW HEALTHY AND PEACEFUL WORLD

Health is a basic human right. We, the people of the earth will not allow this right to be withheld from us any longer. We will not rest until the right to health - particularly the unrestricted access to natural therapies - has become a human right for all people of the world, guaranteed by national and international constitutions.

**I call upon every person on earth:** No matter where you live and what you do you should start building this new world right now! Every living room, every doctor's office or hospital, every school, university, community center, every education text book or movie that promotes natural health is a first step towards creating a healthier world. By constructing this new world we not only eliminate entire diseases but also release billions of dollars in funds that are currently wasted for promoting disease and destruction.

**I call upon the political leaders** to implement natural health as the basis for a prevention-oriented national health care policy. Now that this scientific knowledge is available around the world, you must use it to improve the health of your people. Every country that redirects its health care towards natural health is a quantum leap forward towards a common goal: Health for All by the Year 2020.

There is no time to be lost!

Sincerely,

*Matthias Rath.*

**More information: www.dr-rath-foundation.org**

# Vision for a World
# of Health, Peace and Social Justice

On June 15, 2003, representatives from five continents met in The Hague, the Netherlands and unanimously voted in support of the "Constitution for a World of Peace, Health and Social Justice." This constitution — proclaimed only weeks after the end of the Iraq War — is the beginning of a global health and education campaign to end the "business with disease" and liberate human health from the imposed burden of cardiovascular disease, cancer and many other diseases.

# PEOPLE'S
## CONSTITUTION FOR A WORLD OF

At the beginning of the third millennium mankind stands at the crossroads. On the one hand are the interests of six billion people currently inhabiting our planet - and of all future generations - who wish to live a dignified and healthy life in a peace-ful world. On the other hand is a small corporate interest group denying the whole of mankind these basic human rights for one reason only - financial greed.

In this situation, we, the people of the world, have the choice: we either continue accepting the yoke of those investment industries forcing wars and diseases upon us or we liberate ourselves from these burdens and start building a world determined by the principles of peace, health and social justice.

We, the people of the world, recognize that never before in the course of history have we been more united to preserve peace, to terminate the investment 'business with disease' and to bring to justice those who sacrifice peace and health for corporate gain.

Therefore, we the people from East and West, North and South, from rich and poor countries have decided to create a world of peace, health and social justice for ourselves and generations to come.

As our fundamental rights we proclaim:

**THE RIGHT TO PEACE.** We, the people of the world, are determined to defend our right to peace with all means available. In the age of weapons of mass destruction war is no longer an option for solving international conflicts. We will make sure that those who conduct a war without an explicit mandate by international law will be held responsible and will be brought to justice for their crimes. We will not rest until they are punished - irrespective of economic or political consequences - because we recognize that this is the only way to protect our planet from destruction.

**THE RIGHT TO LIFE.** We, the people of the world, are determined to defend our right to life with all means available. We will not rest until all factors shortening the life span of people on our planet are eliminated. We will fight hunger, malnutrition and other factors already killing millions of inhabitants of our planet each year including infants and children. We will also terminate the 'investment business with disease' as the result of which more people have died prematurely from preventable diseases than in all wars of mankind put together.

## Everyone should support this Agenda!

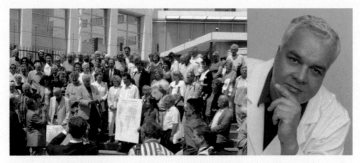

On the same day, I filed a complaint — on behalf of the people of the world — at the United Nation's International Criminal Court in The Hague (ICC) with the goal to forever terminate the promotion of diseases for corporate greed and other crimes against humanity.

# AGENDA
## PEACE, HEALTH AND SOCIAL JUSTICE

**THE RIGHT TO HEALTH.** We, the people of the world, are determined to defend our right to health with all means available. We will make sure that the pharmaceutical 'business with disease' the deliberate promotion of diseases for corporate gain, is outlawed worldwide. We will bring to justice those who deliberately promote diseases and those who withhold live-saving information on natural, non-patentable therapies. In providing health to our communities and in implementing national health care programs we will focus on effective and safe, natural health approaches. The primary goal of any health care strategy is prevention and eradication of diseases.

**THE RIGHT TO SOCIAL JUSTICE.** We, the people of the world, are determined to defend our right to social justice with all means available. We no longer accept that two out of three inhabitants of our planet live in poverty and illiteracy. We will make sure that the resources of the world are redistributed in a way that provides education and a dignified life for every citizen of our planet. To finance this redistribution we will use the financial resources liberated from terminating the multi-trillion dollar 'business with disease' and from decreasing military expenditure.

We recognize that as a first step to reach these goals those corporate interest groups promoting war and disease need to be brought to justice in international courts for sacrificing the lives of mil-lions of people and for committing other crimes against humanity.

Public exposure and punishment of the representatives of these corporate interest groups will remove the last obstacle for the people of the world to terminate the 'Dark Ages of Disease, War and Injustice' and start building a 'New World of Peace, Health and Social Justice'.

On behalf of the people of the world -

*Matthias Rath.*

The Hague, May 2003

**Visit www.dr-rath-health-foundation.org**

# Growing Awareness

Our global information campaign did not go unnoticed. In fact, governmental and private organizations, corporations, universities and other institutions that contacted us via our website are among the "Who's Who" of the world. Following is only a partial list:

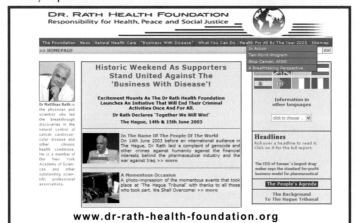

**www.dr-rath-health-foundation.org**

## Government Organizations in:
- Australia
- Belgium
- Brazil
- Canada
- Chile
- Egypt
- Germany
- India
- Italy
- Egypt
- Jordan
- Malaysia
- Netherlands
- Norway
- Poland
- South Africa
- Spain
- Sweden
- Turkey
- USA (Department of Defense)

## Other Institutions:
- Academies of Sciences from:
  Bulgaria, Russia, Sweden
- Development Bank of Singapore
- Dow Jones & Co.
- European Commission
- Ministerio de Salud Chile
- Kaiser Health Insurance (US)
- Karolinska Institute Medical University
- Los Angeles Public Library
- OPEC Fund
- Reuters News Agency
- Royal Communications Jordan
- South African Broadcasting Corp.
- States of California, Florida,
  Georgia, Illinois, Minnesota,
  New Jersey and Texas
- UK National Health Service
- UNO, WHO and UNICEF
- U.S. Centers for Disease Control
- USA Today

# Worldwide Support

## Speaking for millions of supporters around the world:

*"I read your public information in Australia – fantastic work! Congratulations on your integrity!"*
*Australia*

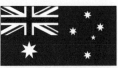

*"I really congratulate you for your courage."*
*Argentina*

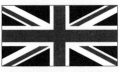

*"I support Dr. Rath in his mission to enlighten the world regarding the truth about pharmaceutical companies."*
*Great Britain*

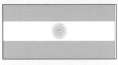

*"I appreciate the work that Dr. Rath is doing to inform me and the world. Whatever we can do to help him affect public and government policy is a step in the right direction."*
*United States*

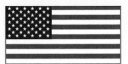

### Corporations:
- Abbott Laboratories
- Bayer
- Boeing
- Chase Manhattan
- Deutsche Bank
- Eli Lilly
- Exxon
- Glaxo Smith Kline Beecham
- Halliburton
- Koch Industries
- Merck
- Microsoft
- Pfizer
- Raytheon Company
- Shell
- Siemens
- Swiss Bank Corporation
- Texaco
- Visa
- Xerox

### Universities:
- Austria: Vienna, Innsbruck
- Brazil:  Buenos Aires
- Canda: McGill
- Cuba: Cienfuegos
- Germany: Heidelberg, Berlin
- France: Grenoble
- India: Madras
- Italy: Bologna, Milan, Rome
- Japan: Nagoya
- Korea: Seoul
- Mexico: National Univ.
- Netherlands: Amsterdam, Rotterdam
- Poland: Warsaw, Krakow
- Singapore: National Univ.
- Spain: Madrid, Seville, Salamanca
- Sweden: School of Economics
- South Africa: Cape Town, Pretoria
- UK: Oxford, Kings, London, Wales
- USA: Stanford, Harvard, Berkeley
  Columbia, Rutgers, Mayo, Yale

# PETITION FOR VITAMIN FREEDOM

Each year, pharmaceutical companies make several hundred billions of dollars solely from worldwide sales of cardiovascular drugs. The natural control of the cardiovascular disease epidemic will lead to the collapse of this market and threaten the existence of this industry.

In its struggle for survival, the pharmaceutical industry has formed a global "pharma-cartel," aiming to block the possibility of eradicating heart disease by natural means. By abusing the World Health Organization's "Codex Alimentarius Commission," the European Parliament and other national and international political institutions, the "pharma-cartel" pursues a worldwide ban on all information about the preventive and therapeutic health benefits of vitamins, minerals and other natural, non-patentable therapies.

In this situation, millions of people worldwide have to protect their own health and lives against the interests of this pharmaceutical investment "business with disease."

Free access to vitamins and unrestricted natural health information worldwide will be the first victory on our way toward the eradication of heart disease and other diseases.

**We demand that our own government and the governments of all other countries:**

- **Abolish all barriers restricting free access to vitamins and other essential nutrients.**

- **Spread the lifesaving information about the health benefits of vitamins and other natural therapies.**

- **Promote the eradication of heart disease and other diseases by all means available.**

**With my signature, I support the "Petition for Vitamin Freedom":**

| Name | Address | Signature |
|------|---------|-----------|

_____

_____

_____

_____

_____

_____

_____

_____

I urge you to support this campaign with your signature. Please also ask your family, friends and colleagues for their support and make this petition the basis of a health initiative in your community.

This petition will continue until we have accomplished our historic goal.

Please return signed copies to my attention at the Dr. Rath Health Foundation, IHZ, Friedrichstrasse 95, D–10117, Berlin. You can also find more information online at **www.dr-rath-health-foundation.org.**

# About the Author

Matthias Rath, M.D. is the world-renowned physician and scientist who led the breakthrough in the natural prevention and treatment of atherosclerosis — the underlying cause of heart attacks and strokes. For this breakthrough, he was awarded the world's first patents for the natural reversal of cardiovascular disease.

Dr. Rath is founder of Cellular Medicine, the fundamentally new scientific understanding that today's most common diseases — including heart disease and cancer — are the consequence of the long-term deficiency of certain vitamins, minerals and other biocatalysts for the metabolism of millions of cells in our bodies.

Dr. Rath's scientific publications have been published in leading international scientific journals, including the American Heart Association's *Arteriosclerosis* and the *Proceedings of the National Academy of Sciences, USA*. His books have been translated into more than 10 languages, and millions of copies have been sold worldwide.

Dr. Rath is the founder and head of an international research and development institute that has as its goal the eradication of today's most common health problems with Cellular Medicine and effective and safe natural therapies.

Dr. Rath's breakthroughs in the effective natural control of heart disease and other conditions have become a threat to the trillion dollar pharmaceutical "business with disease," which is merely based on symptom-oriented, synthetic drugs. As a direct consequence, the drug companies have launched a global campaign to establish "protectionist laws" for their drug markets. Their goal is to ban lifesaving natural health information at the expense of human health and lives.

Dr. Rath's website www.drrath.com is the world's leading source of Cellular Medicine and natural health information.

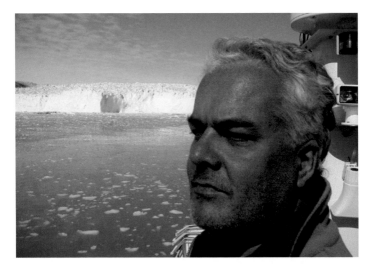

*I find inspiration for my work in nature. While surrounded by the natural world and quiet solitude, I have done my most creative thinking.*

# Acknowledgments

My thanks go to all for without whom the medical breakthrough toward the control of cardiovascular disease would have been delayed by many years: to Dr. Aleksandra Niedzwiecki, my long-time colleague and the entire team of researchers at our Institute, to our employees, to the members of our Health Alliance and to the millions of people and friends worldwide who have been supporting me in this global struggle for the liberation of human health.

My thanks also go to all those who have remained an invaluable source of motivation for me through their skepticism and opposition.

JOURNAL OF APPLIED NUTRITION, VOLUME 48, NUMBER 3          ORIGINAL REPORT

# Nutritional Supplement Program Halts Progression of Early Coronary Atherosclerosis
## Documented by Ultrafast Computed Tomography

Matthias Rath, M.D. and Aleksandra Niedzwiecki, Ph.D.

**ABSTRACT:** The aim of this study was to determine the effect of a defined nutritional supplement program on the natural progression of coronary artery disease. This nutritional supplement program was composed of vitamins, amino acids, minerals, and trace elements, including a combination of essential nutrients patented for use in the prevention and reversal of cardiovascular disease. The study was designed as a prospective intervention before-after trial over a 12-month period and included 55 outpatients ages 44-67 with various stages of coronary heart disease. Changes in the progression of coronary artery calcification before and during the nutritional supplement intervention were determined by Ultrafast Computed Tomography (Ultrafast CT). The natural progression rate of coronary artery calcification before the intervention averaged 44% per year. The progression of coronary artery calcification decreased on average 15% over the course of one year of nutritional supplementation. In a subgroup of patients with early stages of coronary artery disease, a statistically significant decrease occurred, and no further progression of coronary calcification was observed. In individual cases, reversal and complete disappearance of previously existing coronary calcifications were documented. This is the first clinical study documenting the effectiveness of a defined nutritional supplement program in halting early forms of coronary artery disease within one year. The nutritional supplement program tested here should be considered an effective and safe approach for the prevention and adjunct therapy of cardiovascular disease.

Key words: Coronary heart disease, Ultrafast Computed Tomography, nutritional supplements

## INTRODUCTION

According to the World Health Organization, over 12 million people die every year from heart attacks, strokes and other forms of cardiovascular disease.[1] The direct and indirect costs for treatment of cardiovascular disease are the single largest health care expense in every industrialized country of the world. Despite modest success in some countries in lowering the mortality rate from heart attacks and strokes, the cardiovascular epidemic is still expanding on a worldwide scale.

Current concepts of the pathogenesis of cardiovascular disease focus on elevated plasma risk factors damaging the vascular wall and thereby initiating atherogenesis and cardiovascular disease.[2-4] Accordingly, drugs lowering cholesterol and modulating other plasma risk factors have become a predominant therapeutic approach in the prevention of cardiovascular disease.

A new scientific rationale about the initiation of atherosclerosis and cardiovascular disease was proposed by one of us[5,6] It can be summarized as follows: cardiovascular disease is primarily caused by chronic deficiencies of vitamins and other essential nutrients with defined biochemical properties, such as coenzymes, cellular energy carriers, and antioxidants.[7,8] Chronic depletion of these essential nutrients in endothelial and vascular smooth muscle cells impairs their physiological function. For example, chronic ascorbate deficiency, similar to early scurvy, leads to morphological

impairment of the vascular wall and endothelial microlesions, histological hallmarks of early atherosclerosis. [9-11] Consequently, atherosclerotic plaques develop as the result of an overcompensating repair mechanism comprising deposition of systemic plasma factors as well local cellular responses in the vascular wall.[5,6] This repair mechanism is primarily exacerbated at sites of hemodynamic stress, explaining the predominantly local development of atherosclerotic plaques in coronary arteries and myocardial infarction as the most frequent clinical manifestation of cardiovascular disease.

Animal studies have confirmed this scientific rationale resulting in patents for the combination of ascorbate with other essential nutrients in the prevention and treatment of cardiovascular disease.[12] Based on this patented technology, we have developed a nutritional supplement program, which was tested in this study in patients with coronary heart disease.

## SUBJECTS AND METHODS

### Patients

A total of 55 patients, 50 men and 5 women, with documented coronary artery disease assessed by Ultrafast CT were recruited for the study. The inclusion criterion was the availability of a high quality Ultrafast CT scan from a previous visit to the Heart Scan facility in South San Francisco. At the beginning of the study each patient completed a comprehensive questionnaire, which was updated after six months and after 12 months. This questionnaire included medical history, previous cardiac events, and cardiovascular risk factors, as well as individual life style data. Specific questions related to the patients' regular diet, such as strictly vegetarian diet, predominantly fruits and vegetables, predominantly meat, fish or poultry; the daily intake of different vitamins and other essential nutrients; and the frequency of physical exercise by the patient. The laboratory tests available documented a heterogeneous population with respect to plasma cholesterol and triglycerides. About half of the patients were taking different types of prescription medication, including calcium antagonists, nitrates, beta-blockers, and cholesterol-lowering drugs. Before entering the study, the patients were instructed not to change their diet or lifestyle other than adding the nutritional supplement program tested. Any changes were to be documented in their questionnaires. Compliance with the nutritional supplement program was monitored in the questionnaires, through telephone calls and during the control visits.

## Composition and Administration of Nutritional Supplement Program

The following daily dosages of nutritional supplements were taken for a period of one year: Vitamins: Vitamin C 2700 mg, Vitamin E (d-Alpha-Tocopherol) 600 IU, Vitamin A (as Beta-Carotene) 7,500 IU, Vitamin B-1 (Thiamine) 30 mg, Vitamin B-2 (Riboflavin) 30 mg, Vitamin B-3 (as Niacin and Niacinamide) 195 mg, Vitamin B-5 (Pantothenate) 180 mg, Vitamin B-6 (Pyridoxine) 45 mg, Vitamin B-12 (Cyanocobalamin) 90 mcg, Vitamin D (Cholecalciferol) 600 IU. Minerals: Calcium 150 mg, Magnesium 180 mg, Potassium 90 mg, Phosphate 60 mg, Zinc 30 mg, Manganese 6 mg, Copper 1500 mcg, Selenium 90 mcg, Chromium 45 mcg, Molybdenum 18 mcg. Amino acids: L-Proline 450 mg, L-Lysine 450 mg, L-Carnitine 150 mg, L-Arginine 150 mg, L-Cysteine 150 mg. Coenzymes and other nutrients: Folic Acid 390 mcg, Biotin 300 mcg, Inositol 150 mg, Coenzyme Q-10 30 mg, Pycnogenol 30 mg, and Citrus Bioflavonoids 450 mg. Further information at: www.drrath.com

## Monitoring of Coronary Artery Disease

The extent of coronary calcification was measured non-invasively with an Imatron C-100 Ultrafast CT scanner in the high-resolution volume mode, using a 100-millisecond exposure time. ECG triggering was used so that each image was obtained at the same point in the diastole, corresponding to 80% of the RR interval. In each scan, 30 consecutive images were obtained at 3mm intervals beginning 1 cm below the carina and progressing caudally to include the entire length of the coronary arteries. The scans at study entry and after 6 and 12 months of the study included a second scan sequence of 30 images at 3 mm intervals across the entire heart. The 30 images of the second scan were taken between the 3 mm intervals of the first scan resulting in a scanning of the heart at an interval of 1.5 mm. Total radiation exposure using this technique was <1rad per patient (<.01Gy).

The scan threshold was set at 130 Hounsfield units (Hu) for identification of calcified lesions. The minimum area to differentiate calcified lesions from CT artifact was 0.68 mm$^2$. The lesion score, also designated Coronary Artery Scanning (CAS) score, was calculated by multiplying the lesion area by a density factor derived from the maximal Hounsfield unit within this area.[13] The density factor was assigned in the following way: 1 for lesions with a maximal density with 130-199 Hu, 2 for lesions with 200-299 Hu, 3 for lesions with 300-399 Hu and 4 for lesions > 400 Hu. The total calcium areas and CAS scores of each Ultrafast CT scan were determined by summing individual lesion areas or scores from the left main, left anterior descending, circumflex, and right coronary artery.

Several studies have confirmed an excellent correlation of the extent of coronary artery disease as assessed by Ultrafast CT scanning when compared to angiographic and histomorphometric methods.[13-15] Considering the accuracy and the non-invasive approach, Ultrafast CT was the method of choice for an intervention study that included early, asymptomatic stages of coronary artery disease.

**Table 1:** Clinical data of study participants from patient protocol at study onset

|  |  | All Patients (n=55) | | Patients With Starting Coronary Sclerosis (n=21) | |
|---|---|---|---|---|---|
| Age: | 40-49 | 5 | (9%) | 4 | (8%) |
|  | 50-59 | 24 | (44%) | 8 | (40%) |
|  | 60-69 | 26 | (47%) | 9 | (52%) |
| Smoker | | 4 | (7%) | 1 | (5%) |
| Ex-smoker | | 36 | (65%) | 12 | (57%) |
| Diabetic | | 4 | (7%) | 0 | (0%) |
| Pancreas failure | | 3 | (5%) | 1 | (5%) |
| Heart attack | | 5 | (9%) | 0 | (0%) |
| Angioplasty, balloon catheter | | 2 | (4%) | 1 | (5%) |
| Use of medications | | 27 | (49%) | 7 | (33%) |
| Use of vitamins | | 36 | (65%) | 15 | (71%) |

299

## Statistical Analysis

The growth rate of coronary calcifications was calculated as the quotient of the differences in the calcification areas or CAS scores between two scans divided by the months between these scans according to the formula (Area2-Area1):(Date2-Date1), or (CAS score 2-CAS score1):(Date2-Date1) respectively. The data were analyzed using standard formulas for means, medians, and standard error of the means (SEM). Pearson's correlation coefficient was used to determine the association between continuous variables. One tailed Student t-test was used to analyze differences between mean values, with a significance defined at <0.5. Progression of calcification was predicted by linear extrapolation. The distribution of the growth rate of CAS scores was described by a smooth curve resulting from a third order polynominal fit ($y = a + bx^3$, where $a = 0.9352959$, $b = 8.8235 \times 10^{-5}$).

## RESULTS

The aim of this study was to determine the effect of a defined nutritional supplement program on the natural progression of coronary artery calcification particularly in its initial stages as measured by Ultrafast CT. We therefore evaluated the results of the entire study group (n=55) and of a subgroup of 21 patients with early coronary artery calcification, as defined by a CAS score of <100.

Table 2 separately lists the characteristics of the study population assessed by the questionnaire for all patients and for a subgroup with early coronary artery disease.

This is the first intervention study using Imatron's Ultrafast CT technology. One of the first aims of this

study was to determine the rate of natural progression of coronary calcium deposits *in situ*, without the intervention of the nutritional supplement program. Figure 1 shows the distribution of the monthly progression of calcifications in the coronary arteries of all 55 patients in relation to their CAS score at study entry.

We found that the higher the CAS score was initially, without intervention, the faster the coronary calcification progressed. Accordingly, the average monthly growth rate of coronary calcifications ranged from 1 CAS score per month in patients with early coronary heart disease to more than 15 CAS score per month in patients with advanced stages of coronary calcifications. The growth pattern of coronary calcifications can be described as a third order polynomial fit curve. The exponential shape of this curve signifies a first quantification of the aggressive nature of coronary atherosclerosis and emphasizes the importance of early intervention.

The changes in the natural progression rate of coronary artery calcification before the nutritional supplement program (-NS) and after one year on this program (+NS) are shown in Figure 2. The results are presented separately for the calcified area and the CAS score.

As presented in Figure 2a the average monthly growth of calcified areas for all 55 patients decreased from 1.24 mm²/month (SEM +/- 0.3) before the nutritional supplement program (-NS) to 1.05 mm²/month (+/- 0.2) after one year on this program (+NS). For patients with early coronary artery disease (Figure 2b), the average monthly growth of the calcified area decreased from 0.49 mm²/month (+/- 0.16) before taking the nutritional supplements (-NS) to 0.28 mm²/month (+/- 0.09) after one year on this program (+NS).

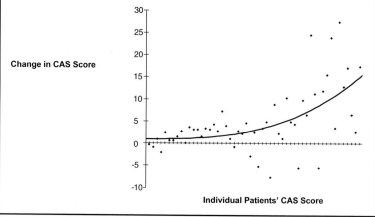

**Figure 1.** Distribution of monthly increase in CAS scores in relation to CAS scores at study entry. The data represent all 55 patients individually. The calcification rate distribution pattern can be described by the polynominal curve: $y = a + bx^3$, where $a = 0.9352959$, $b = 8.8235 \times 10^{-5}$.

As shown in Figure 2c the average monthly changes in the total CAS score (calcified area X density of calcium deposits) for all 55 patients had decreased after one year on the nutritional supplement program by 11%, from 4.8 CAS score/month (SEM +/-0.97) before the program (-NS) to 4.27 CAS score /month(+/- 0.87) (+NS). In patients with early coronary artery disease (Figure 2d) the average monthly growth of the total CAS score decreased during the same time by as much as 65%, from 1.85 CAS score /month (+/-0.49) before the nutritional supplement program (-NS) to 0.65 CAS score /month (+/- 0.36) on this program (+NS). The slow-down of the progression of coronary calcification during this nutritional supplement intervention for CAS scores of patients with early coronary artery disease was statistically significant (p<0.05)(Figure 2d). For the other three sets of data the decrease of coronary calcifications with the nutritional supplement program was evident; however, largely due to the wide range of calcification values at study entry reflecting the different stages of coronary artery disease, it did not reach statistical significance.

It is noteworthy that the decrease in the CAS scores during intervention with nutritional supplements were more pronounced than for the calcified areas. This indicates a decrease in the density of calcium in addition to a reduction in the area of coronary calcium deposits during nutritional supplement intervention.

Ultrafast CT scans at the beginning of the study and after 12 months on the nutritional supplement program, were complemented by a control scan after 6 months, allowing for additional insight into the time required for the nutritional supplements to exert their therapeutic effect. This additional evaluation was particularly important for early forms of coronary artery disease, because any therapeutic approach that can halt progression of early coronary calcification would ultimately prevent myocardial infarctions.

Figure 3 shows the average coronary calcification areas (Figure 3a) and total CAS scores (Figure 3b) for patients with early coronary artery disease measured during different scanning dates before and during the course of the study. The actual coronary calcification values for areas and total CAS scores during nutritional supplement intervention are compared to the predicted values obtained from linear extrapolation of the growth rate without intervention. The letters A to D mark the different time points at which Ultrafast CT scans were performed. AB represents the changes in coronary calcification before intervention with nutritional supplement for the areas (Figure 3a) and CAS scores (Figure 3b). Accordingly, BC represents calcification changes during the first six months on the nutritional supplement program and CD changes during the second six months on the program. The calculated progression rate for coronary calcifications without therapeutic intervention by the nutritional supplement program is

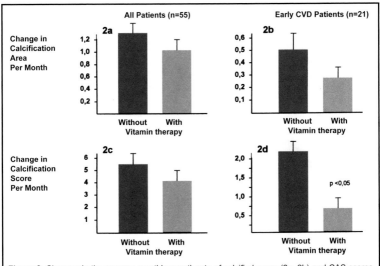

**Figure 2.** Changes in the average monthly growth rate of calcified areas (2a, 2b) and CAS scores (2c,2d) in all study participants (n=55) and in a subgroup of patients with initial stages of coronary calcifications (CAS score<100, n=21), before nutritional supplement intervention (-NS) and after one year of intervention (+NS). Data are mean +/- SEM, asterisk indicates significance at p < 0.05 (one tailed t-test).

301

marked by a dotted line (B through F).

As seen in Figure 3a without the nutritional supplement program, the average area of coronary calcifications in patients with early coronary artery disease increased from 17.62 mm² (+/- 1.0) at time point A to 23.05 mm² (+/- 1.8) at time point B. Thus, the annual extension of calcified areas without intervention was assessed with 31 %. At this progression rate, the average calcified area would reach 26.3 mm² after six months (point E) and 29.8 mm² after twelve months (point F). The nutritional supplement intervention, resulted in an average calcified area of 25.2 mm2 (+/- 2.2) after six months and of 27.0 mm2 (+/-1.7) after 12 months, reflecting a 10% decrease compared to the predicted value.

Analogous observations were made for the total CAS before and during the nutritional supplement program. Figure 3.b shows that the CAS score before the nutritional supplement program increased by 44% per year, from 45.8 (+/- 3.2) (point A) to 65.9 mm2 (+/- 5.2) (point B). At this progression rate the total CAS score, without the nutritional supplement program, would reach an average of 77.9 after six months (point E) and of 91 (point F) after 12 months. In contrast to this trend the actual CAS score values measured with the nutritional supplement program were 75.8 (+/-6.2) after 6 months (point C) and 78.1 (+/-5.1) after 12 months (point D). Thus, the progression of coronary calcification as determined by the total CAS scores decreased significantly during the second six months of nutritional supplement intervention (CD). The total score after twelve months on the nutritional supplement program was only 3% higher than after six months (CD), as compared to the projected increase of 17% (EF), indicating that during the second six months on the nutri-

tional supplement program the process of coronary calcification has practically stopped.

Figure 4 shows the actual Ultrafast CT scans of a 51-year-old patient with early, asymptomatic, coronary artery disease. The patients' first Ultrafast CT scan was performed in 1993 as part of an annual routine checkup. The scan film revealed small calcifications in the left anterior descendent coronary artery as well as in the right coronary artery. The second CT scan was performed one year later at which time the initial calcium deposits had further increased. Figure 4a shows two Ultrafast CT scan images taken before the nutritional supplement program.

Subsequently, the patient started on the nutritional supplement program. About one year later the patient received a control scan. At this time point, coronary calcifications were not found (Figure 4b.), indicating the natural reversal of coronary artery disease.

## DISCUSSION

This is the first study that provides quantifiable data from *in situ* measurements about the natural progression rate of coronary artery disease. Although atherosclerotic plaques have a complex histomorphological composition, calcium dispersion within these plaques has been shown to be an excellent marker for their advancement.[11,13] Our study determined that the calcified vascular areas expand at a rate between 5 mm2 (early atherosclerotic lesions) and 40 mm2 (advanced atherosclerotic lesions). Before the nutritional supplement program the average annual increase of total coronary calcification was 44% (Figure 1). Considering

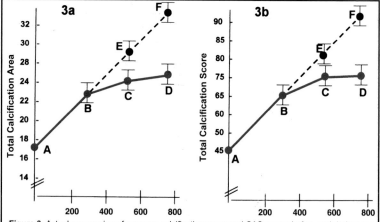

**Figure 3.** Actual progression of coronary calcification areas and CAS scores before and during one year of nutritional supplement intervention in a subgroup of patients with initial stages of coronary calcification (CAS <100), compared to calculated progression without intervention (dotted line). Each data point represents the mean value +/- SEM.

the exponential increase of coronary calcification, it is evident that the control of cardiovascular disease has to focus on early diagnosis and early intervention.

Today, the diagnostic assessment of individual cardiovascular risk is largely confined to the measurement of plasma cholesterol and other risk factors with little correlation to the extent of atherosclerotic plaques. More accurate methods, such as coronary angiography, are confined to advanced, symptomatic, stages of coronary artery disease. Ultrafast CT provides the diagnostic option to quantify coronary artery disease non-invasively in its early stages.[14,15]

The most important finding of this study is that coronary artery disease can be effectively prevented and treated by natural means. This nutritional supplement program was able to decrease the progression of coronary artery disease within the relatively short time of one year, irrespective of the stage of this disease. Most significantly, in patients with early coronary calcifications this nutritional supplement program was able to essentially stop its further progression. In individual cases with small calcified deposits, nutritional supplement intervention led to their complete disappearance (Figure 4).

We postulate that the nutritional supplement program tested in this study initiates the reconstitution of the vascular wall. Restructuring of the vascular matrix is facilitated by several nutrients tested, such as ascorbate (vitamin C), pyridoxine (vitamin B-6), L-lysine, and L-proline, as well as the trace element copper. Ascorbate is essential for the synthesis and hydroxylation of collagen and other matrix components,[16-18] and can be directly and indirectly involved in a variety of regulatory mechanisms in the vascular wall from cell differen-

tiation to distribution of growth factors.[19,20] Pyridoxine and copper are essential for the proper cross-linking of matrix components.[8] L-lysine and L-proline are important substrates for the biosynthesis of matrix proteins; they also competitively inhibit the binding of lipoprotein(a) to the vascular matrix, facilitating the release of lipoprotein(a) and other lipoproteins from the vascular wall.[5,12,21] Ascorbate and -tocopherol have been shown to inhibit the proliferation of vascular smooth muscle cells.[22-24] Moreover, tocopherols, beta-carotene, ascorbate, selenium and other antioxidants scavenge free radicals and protect plasma constituents, as well as vascular tissue, from oxidative damage.[25,26] In addition, nicotinate, riboflavin, pantothenate, carnitine, coenzyme Q-10, as well as many minerals and trace elements, function as cellular cofactors in form of NADH, NADPH, FADH, Coenzyme A and other cellular energy carriers.[8] The results of this study confirm that maintaining the integrity and physiological function of the vascular wall is the key therapeutic target in controlling cardiovascular disease. This also corroborates early angiographic findings that supplemental vitamin C may halt the progression of atherosclerosis in femoral arteries.[27]

These conclusions are even more relevant since deficiencies of essential nutrients are common.[28,29] Moreover, many epidemiological and clinical studies have already documented the benefits of individual nutrients in the prevention of cardiovascular disease.[30-35] Compared to the high dosages of vitamins used in some of these studies the amounts of nutrients used in this study are moderate, indicating the synergistic effect of this program.

In this context, it seems appropriate to critically review some of the approaches currently used in the

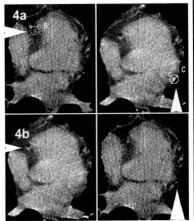

**Figure 4.** Ultrafast CT scan images of a 50-year-old patient with asymptomatic coronary artery disease before the nutritional supplement program (top row) and approximately one year later (bottom row). Calcium deposits in the left descending coronary artery and in the right coronary artery are visible as white areas.

primary and secondary prevention of cardiovascular disease, including the extensive use of cholesterol-lowering drugs. An intervention study including lovastatin was performed with a highly selected group of hyperlipidemic patients, representing only an extremely narrow fraction of a normal population.[36] More recently, the reduction of myocardial infarctions and other cardiac events in patients taking simvastatin, led to recommendations for its long-term use even by normolipidemic patients.[37] However, because of their potential side-effects, the recommended use of these drugs has now been restricted to patients at high short-term risk for coronary heart disease.[38]

Similarly, certain natural approaches to prevention of cardiovascular disease deserve a critical review. A program of rigorous diet and exercise program claims to be able to reverse coronary heart disease.[39] However, the published study does not provide compelling evidence documenting the regression of coronary atherosclerosis. Thus, the improved myocardial perfusion shown in that study, was likely the result of the physical training program, leading to an increased ventricular ejection fraction and an increased coronary perfusion pressure.

Considering the urgent need for effective and safe public health measures towards the control of cardiovascular disease, the validity of this study is of particular importance. In light of this, the following study elements are noteworthy:

1. The patients in this study served as their own controls before and during nutritional supplement intervention, thereby minimizing undesired co-variables such as age, gender, genetic predisposition, diet or medication.

2. Ultrafast CT has been extensively validated to assess the degree of coronary atherosclerosis, and it allowed quantification of coronary atherosclerotic plaques *in situ*.[13-15] This diagnostic technique also minimizes errors as they occur in angiography studies in which vasospasms, formation or lysis of thrombi, and other events cannot be differentiated from progression or regression of atherosclerotic plaques. Moreover, Ultrafast CT provides valuable information about the morphological changes during progression and regression of atherosclerotic plaques, by quantifying not only the area of coronary calcifications but also their density. Furthermore, the automatic CT measurements of coronary calcifications eliminates human error in the evaluation of the data.

In summary, the results of this study imply that coronary heart disease is a preventable and essentially reversible condition. This study documents that coronary artery disease could be halted in its early stages by following this nutritional supplement program. These results were achieved within one year, suggesting that additional therapeutic benefits in patients with advanced coronary artery disease can be obtained by an extended use of this program. The continuation of this study is currently under way to document these effects. This nutritional supplement program signifies an effective and safe approach for the prevention and adjunct therapy of cardiovascular disease. This study should encourage public health policy makers and health care providers to redefine health strategies towards the control of cardiovascular disease.

## ACKNOWLEDGEMENTS

We are grateful to Jeffrey Kamradt for his help in coordinating this study. Douglas Boyd, Ph.D., Lew Meyer, Ph.D. from Imatron/HeartScan., South San Francisco, for helping to plan the study and providing the HeartScan facility; Lauranne Cox, Susan Brody, and Tom Caruso for their collaboration in conducting the heart scans. Dr. Roger Barth and Bernard Murphy for their assistance in planning the study, as well as to Martha Best for her secretarial assistance.

## REFERENCES

1. World Health Statistics, World Health Organization, Geneva, 1994.

2. Brown MS, Goldstein JL. How LDL receptors influence cholesterol and atherosclerosis. *Scientific American* 1984;251:58-66.

3. Steinberg D, Parthasarathy S, Carew TE, Witztum JL. Modifications of low-density lipoprotein that increase its atherogenicity. *N Engl J Med.* 1989;320:915-924.

4. Ross R. The pathogenesis of atherosclerosis-an update. *N Engl J Med.* 1986;314:488-500.

5. Rath M, Pauling L. A unified theory of human cardiovascular disease leading the way to the abolition of this diseases as a cause for human mortality. *J Ortho Med.* 1992;7:5-15.

6. Rath M, Pauling L. Solution to the puzzle of human cardiovascular disease: Its primary cause is ascorbate deficiency, leading to the deposition of lipoprotein(a) and fibrinogen/fibrin in the vascular wall. *J Ortho Med.* 1991;6:125-134.

7. Rath M. Reducing the risk for cardiovascular disease with nutritional supplements. *J Ortho Med* 1992;3:1-6.

8. Stryer L. *Biochemistry*, 3rd ed. New York: W.H.Freeman and Company; 1988.

9. Stary HC. Evolution and progression of atherosclerotic lesions in coronary arteries of children and young adults. *Atherosclerosis (Suppl.)* 1989;9:I-19-I-32.

10. Constantinides P. The role of arterial wall injury in atherogenesis and arterial thrombogenesis. *Zentralbl allg Pathol pathol Anat.* 1989;135:517-530.

11. Stolman JM, Goldman HM, Gould BS. Ascorbic acid in blood vessels. *Arch Pathol.* 1961;72:59-68.

12. US Patent #5,278,189

13. Agatston AS, Janowitz WR, Kaplan G, Gasso J, Hildner F, Viamonte M. Ultrafast computed tomography—detected coronary calcium reflects the angiographic extent of coronary arterial atherosclerosis.

*Am J Cardiology.* 1994;74:1272-1274.

14. Budoff MJ, Georgiou D, Brody A, et al. Ultrafast computed tomography as a diagnostic modality in the detection of coronary artery disease. *Circulation.* 1996; 93:898-904.

15. Mautner SI, Mautner GC, Froehlich J, et al. Coronary artery disease: prediction with in vitro electron beam CT. *Radiology.* 1994;192:625-630.

16. Murad S, Grove D, Lindberg KA, Reynolds G, Sivarajah A, Pinnell SR. Regulation of collagen synthesis by ascorbic acid. *Proc Natl Acad Sci.* 1981;78:2879-2882.

17. De Clerck YA, Jones PA. The effect of ascorbic acid on the nature and production of collagen and elastin by rat smooth muscle cells. *Biochem J.* 1980;186:217-225.

18. Schwartz E, Bienkowski RS, Coltoff-Schiller B, Goldfisher S, Blumenfeld OO. Changes in the components of extracellular matrix and in growth properties of cultured aortic smooth muscle cells upon ascorbate feeding. *J Cell Biol.* 1982;92:462-470.

19. Francheschi RT. The role of ascorbic acid in mesenchymal differentiation. *Nutr Rev.* 1992;50:65-70.

20. Dozin B, Quatro R, Campanile g, Cancedda R. In vitro differentiation of mouse embryo chondrocytes: requirement for ascorbic acid. *Eur J Cell Biol.* 1992;58:390-394.

21. Trieu VN, Zioncheck TF, Lawn RM, McConathy WJ. Interaction of apolipoprotein(a) with apolipoprotein B-containing lipoproteins. *J Biol Chem.* 1991; 226:5480-5485.

22. Boscoboinik D, Szewczyk A, Hensey C, Azzi A. Inhibition of cell proliferation by -tocopherol. Role of protein kinase C. *J Biol Chem.* 1991; 266:6188-6194.

23. Ivanov V, Niedzwiecki A. Direct and extracellular matrix mediated effects of ascorbate on vascular smooth muscle cells proliferation. *24th AAA (Age) and 9th Am Coll Clin Gerontol Meeting*, Washington DC, 1994; Oct 14-18.

24. Nunes GL, Sgoutas DS, Redden RA, Sigman SR, Gravanis MB, King SB, Berk BC. Combination of vitamins C and E alters the response to coronary balloon injury in the pig. *Arteriosclerosis, Thrombosis and Vascular Biology.* 1995; 15:156-165.

25. Retsky KL, Freeman MW, Frei B. Ascorbic acid oxidation product(s) protect human low density lipoprotein against atherogenic modification. Antirather than prooxidant activity of vitamin C in the presence of transition metal ions. *J Biol Chem.* 1993;268:1304-1309.

26. Sies H, Stahl W. Vitamins E and C, -carotene and other carotenoids as antioxidants. *Am J Clin Nutr.* 1995;62(Suppl);1315S-1321S.

27. Willis GC, Light AW, Gow WS. Serial arteriography in atherosclerosis. *Can Med Ass J.* 1954;71:562-568.

28. Levine M, Contry-Caritilena C, Wang Y, et al. Vitamin C pharmacokinetics in healthy volunteers: Evidence for a recommended daily allowance. *Proc Natl Acad Sci.* 1996;93:3704-3709.

29. Naurath HJ, Joosten E, Riezler R. Effects of vitamin B12, folate, and vitamin B6 supplements in elderly people with normal serum vitamin concentrations. *The Lancet.* 1995;346:85-89.

30. Enstrom JE, Kanim LE, Klein MA. Vitamin C intake and mortality among a sample of the United States population. *Epidemiology.* 1992; 3: 194-202.

31. Riemersma RA, Wood DA, Macintyre CCA, Elton RA, Gey KF, Oliver MF. Risk of angina pectoris and plasma concentrations of vitamin A, C, and E and carotene. *The Lancet.* 1991;337:1-5.

32. Hodis HN, Mack WJ, LaBree L, et al. Serial coronary angiographic evidence that antioxidant vitamin intake reduces progression of coronary artery atherosclerosis. *JAMA.* 1995; 273:1849-1854.

33. Morrison HI, Schaubel D, Desmeules M, Wigle DT. Serum folate and risk of fatal coronary heart disease. *JAMA.* 1996; 275:1893-1896.

34. Stephens NG, Parsons A, Schofield PM, et al. Randomised controlled trial of vitamin E in patients with coronary disease: Cambridge Heart Antioxidant Study (CHAOS). *The Lancet.* 1996;347:781-786.

35. Heitzer T, Just H, Münzel T. Antioxidant vitamin C improves endothelial dysfunction in chronic smokers. *Am Heart Assoc.* 1996;comm:6-9.

36. Brown BG, Albers JJ, Fisher LD, Schafer SM, Lin J-T, *et al.* Regression of coronary artery disease as a result of intensive lipid-lowering therapy in men with high levels of apolipoprotein B. *N Engl J Med.* 1990;323:1289-1298.

37. Scandinavian Simvastatin Survival Study Group. Randomised trial of cholesterol lowering in 4444 patients with coronary heart disease: the Scandinavian Simvastatin Survival Study (4S). *The Lancet* 1994;344:1383-1389.

38. Newman TB, Hulley SB. Carcinogenicity of lipid-lowering drugs. *JAMA.* 1996;275:55-60.

39. Gould KL, Ornish D, Scherwitz L, et al. Changes in myocardial perfusion abnormalities by positron emission tomography after long-term, intense risk factor modification. *JAMA* 1995;274:894-901.

# References

**The following comprehensive list of references is compiled to document the broad support nutritional and Cellular Medicine already has. You will find these publications in larger public libraries and in the library of any medical school.**

Armstrong VW, Cremer P, Eberle E, et. al. (1986) The association between serum Lp(a) concentrations and angiographically assessed coronary atherosclerosis. Dependence on serum LDL-levels. *Atherosclerosis* 62: 249-257.

Altschul R, Hoffer A, Stephen JD. (1955) Influence of nicotinic acid on serum cholesterol in man. *Archives of Biochemistry and Biophysics* 54: 558-559.

Aulinskas TH, Van der Westhuyzen DR, Coetzee GA. (1983) Ascorbate increases the number of low-density lipoprotein receptors in cultured arterial smooth muscle cells. *Atherosclerosis* 47: 159-171.

Avogaro P, Bon GB, Fusello M. (1983) Effect of pantethine on lipids, lipoproteins and apolipoproteins in man. *Current Therapeutic Research* 33: 488-493.

Bates CJ, Mandal AR, Cole TJ. (1977) HDL. Cholesterol and vitamin C status. *The Lancet* 3:611.

Beamish R. (1993) Vitamin E - then and now. *Canadian Journal of Cardiology* 9: 29-31.

Beisiegel U, Niendorf A, Wolf K, Reblin T, Rath M. (1990) Lipoprotein (a) in the arterial wall. *European Heart Journal* 11 (Supplement E): 174-183.

Bendich A. (1992) Safety issues regarding the use of vitamin supplements. *Annals of the New York Academy of Sciences* 669: 300-310.

Berg K. (1963) A new serum type system in man - the Lp system. *Acta Pathologica Scandinavia* 59: 369-382.

Blumberg A, Hanck A, Sandner G. (1983) Vitamin nutrition in patients on continuous ambulatory peritoneal dialysis (CAPD). *Clinical Nephrology* 20: 244-250.

Braunwald E. (Editor) (1992) *Heart Disease – A Textbook of Cardiovascular Medicine.* W.B. Saunders & Company, Philadelphia.

Briggs M, Briggs M. (1972) Vitamin C requirements and oral contraceptives. *Nature* 238: 277.

Carlson LA, Hamsten A, Asplund A. (1989). Pronounced lowering of serum levels of lipoprotein Lp(a) in hyperlipidemic subjects treated with nicotinic acid. *Journal of Internal Medicine (England)* 226: 271-276.

Cherchi A, Lai C, Angelino F, et. al. (1985) Effects of L-carnitine on exercise tolerance in chronic stable angina: a multicenter, double-blind, randomized, placebo controlled crossover study. *Int J Clin Pharmacol Ther Toxicol* 23(10): 569-572.

Chow CK, Changchit C, Bridges RBI, Rein SR, Humble J, Turk J. (1986) Lower levels of vitamin C and carotenes in plasma of cigarette smokers. *Journal of the American College of Nutrition* 5: 305-312.

Clemetson CAB. (1989) *Vitamin C, Volume I-III.* CRC Press Inc., Florida.

Cushing GL, Gaubatz JW, Nave ML, Burdick BJ, Bocan TMA, Guyton JR, Weilbaecher D, DeBakey ME, Lawrie GM, Morrisett JD. (1989) Quantitation and localization of lipoprotein (a) and B in coronary artery bypass vein grafts resected at re-operation. *Arteriosclerosis* 9: 593-603.

Dahlen GH, Guyton JR, Attar M, Farmer JA, Kautz JA, Gotto AM, Jr. (1986) Association of levels of lipoprotein LP(a), plasma lipids, and other lipoproteins with coronary artery disease documented by angiography. *Circulation* 74: 758-765.

DeMaio SJ, King SB, Lembo NJ, Roubin GS, Hearn JA, Bhagavan HN, Sgoutas DS. (1992) Vitamin E supplementation, plasma lipids and incidence of restenosis after percutaneous transluminal coronary angioplasty (PTCA). *Journal of the American College of Nutrition* 11: 68-73.

Dice JF, Daniel CW. (1973) The hypoglycemic effect of ascorbic acid in a juvenile-onset diabetic. *International Research Communications System* 1: 41.

307

Digiesi V. (1992) Mechanism of action of coenzyme Q10 in essential hypertension. *Current Therapeutic Research* 51: 668-672.

Emmert D, Irchner J. (1999) The role of vitamin E in the prevention of heart disease. *Archives of Family Medicine* 8: 537-542.

England M. (1992) Magnesium administration and dysrhythmias after cardiac surgery: A placebo-controlled, double-blind randomized trial. *Journal of the American Medical Association* 268: 2395-2402.

Enstrom JE, Kanim LE, Klein MA. (1992) Vitamin C intake and mortality among a sample of the United States population. *Epidemiology* 3: 194-202.

Ferrari R, Cucchini, Visioli O. (1984) The metabolical effects of L-carnitine in angina pectoris. *International Journal of Cardiology* 5: 213-216.

Folkers K, Yamamura Y. (Editors) (1976, 1979, 1981, 1984, 1986) *Biomedical and Clinical Aspects of Coenzyme Q, Volume 1-5.* Elsevier Science Publishers, New York.

Folkers K, Vadhanavikit S, Mortensen SA. (1985) Biochemical rationale and myocardial tissue data on the effective therapy of cardiomyopathy with coenzyme Q10. *Proceedings of the National Academy of Sciences, USA* 82: 901-904.

Folkers K, Langsjoen P, Willis R, Richardson P, Xia LJ, Ye CQ, Tamagawa H. (1990) Lovastatin decreases coenzyme Q-10 levels in humans. *Proceedings of the National Academy of Sciences, USA* 87: 8931-8934.

Gaby SK, Bendich A, Singh VN, Machlin LJ (1991) *Vitamin intake and health.* Marcel Dekker Inc., New York.

Gaddi A, Descovich GC, Noseda G, Fragiacomo C, Colombo L, Craveri A, Montanari G, Sirtori CR. (1984) Controlled evaluation of pantethine, a natural hypolipidemic compound, in patients with different forms of hyperlipoproteinemia. *Atherosclerosis* 5: 73-83.

Galeone F, Scalabrino A, Giuntoli F, Birindelli A, Panigada G, Rossi, Saba P. (1983) The lipid-lowering effect of pantethine in hyperlipidemic patients: A clinical investigation. *Current Therapeutic Research* 34: 383-390.

Genest J Jr., Jenner JL, McNamara JR, Ordovas JM, Silberman SR, Wilson PWF, Schaefer EJ. (1991) Prevalence of lipoprotein (a) Lp(a) excess in coronary artery disease. *American Journal of Cardiology* 67: 1039-1045.

Gerster H. (1991) Potential role of beta-carotene in the prevention of cardiovascular disease. *International Journal of Vitamin and Nutrition Research* 61: 277-291.

Gey KF, Stahelin HB, Puska P, Evans A. (1987)Relationship of plasma level of vitamin C to mortality from ischemic heart disease. *Ann NY Acad Sci* 498: 110-123.

Gey KF, Puska P, Jordan P, Moser UK. (1991) Inverse correlation between plasma vitamin E and mortality from ischemic heart disease in cross-cultural epidemiology. *American Journal of Clinical Nutrition* 53: 326, Supplement.

Ghidini O, Azzurro M, Vita A, Sartori G. (1988) Evaluation of the therapeutic efficacy of L-carnitine in congestive heart failure. *International Journal of Clinical Pharmacology, Therapy and Toxicology* 26: 217-220.

Ginter E. (1973) Cholesterol: Vitamin C controls its transformation into bile acids. *Science* 179: 702.

Ginter E. (1978) Marginal vitamin C deficiency, lipid metabolism, and atherosclerosis. *Lipid Research* 16: 216-220.

Ginter E. (1991) Vitamin C deficiency, cholesterol metabolism, and atherosclerosis. *Journal of Orthomolecular Medicine* 6: 166-173.

Guraker A, Hoeg JM, Kostner G, Papadopoulos NM, Brewer HB Jr. (1985) Levels of lipoprotein Lp(a) decline with neomycin and niacin treatment. *Atherosclerosis* 57: 293-301.

Halliwell B, Gutteridge JMC (1985) *Free Radicals in Biology and Medicine.* Oxford University Press, London, New York, Toronto.

Harwood HJ Jr, Greene YJ, Stacpoole PW (1986) Inhibition of human leucocyte 3-hydroxy-3-methylglutaryl coenzyme A reductase activity by ascorbic acid. An effect mediated by the free radical monodehydro-ascorbate. *Journal of Biological Chemistry* 261: 7127-7135.

Hearn JA, Donohue BC, Ba'albaki H, Douglas JS, King SBIII, Lembo NJ, Roubin JS, Sgoutas DS. (1992) Usefulness of serum lipoprotein (a) as a predictor of restenosis after percutaneous transluminal coronary angioplasty. *The American Journal of Cardiology* 68: 736-739.

Hennekens, C. See: Rimm EB (1993) and Stampfer (1993).

Hermann WJ JR, Ward K, Faucett J. (1979) The effect of tocopherol on high-density lipoprotein cholesterol. *American Journal of Clinical Pathology* 72: 848-852.

Hemilä H. (1992) Vitamin C and plasma cholesterol. In: *Critical Reviews in Food Science and Nutrition* 32 (1): 33-57. CRC Press Inc., Florida.

Hoff HF, Beck GJ, Skibinski CI, Jürgens G, O'Neil J, Kramer J, Lytle B. (1988) Serum Lp(a) level as a predictor of vein graft stenosis after coronary artery bypass surgery in patients. *Circulation* 77: 1238-1244.

Ivanov V, Ivanova S, Niedzwiecki A. (1997) Ascorbate affects proliferation of guinea pigs vascular smooth muscle cells by direct and extracellular matrix mediated effects. *J Mol Cell Cardiol* 29: 3293-3303.

Iseri LT. (1986) Magnesium and cardiac arrhythmias. *Magnesium* 5: 111-126.

Iseri LT, French JH. (1984) Magnesium: Nature's physiologic calcium blocker. *American Heart Journal* 108: 188-193.

Jacques PF, Hartz SC, McGandy RB, Jacob RA, Russell RM. (1987) Ascorbic acid, HDL, and total plasma cholesterol in the elderly. *Journal of the American College of Nutrition* 6: 169-174.

Kamikawa T, Kobayashi A, Emaciate T, Hayashi H, Yamazaki N. (1985) Effects of coenzyme Q-10 on exercise tolerance in chronic stable angina pectoris. *American Journal of Cardiology* 56: 247-251.

Koh ET (1984) Effect of Vitamin C on blood parameters of hypertensive subjects. *Oklahoma State Medical Association Journal* 77: 177-182.

Korbut R. (1993) Effect of L-arginine on plasminogen-activator inhibitor in hypertensive patients with hypercholesterolemia. *New England Journal of Medicine* 328 [4]: 287-288.

Kostner GM, Avogaro P, Cazzolato G, Marth E, Bittolo-Bon G, Qunici GB. (1981) Lipoprotein Lp(a) and the risk for myocardial infarction. *Atherosclerosis* 38: 51-61.

Kurl S, Tuomainen TP, Laukkanen JA, et. al. (2002) Plasma vitamin C modifies the association between hypertension and risk of stroke. *Stroke* 33(6): 1568-73.

Langsjoen PH, Folkers K, Lyson K, Muratsu K, Lyson T, Langsjoen P. (1988) Effective and safe therapy with coenzyme Q10 for cardiomyopathy. *Klinische Wochenschrift* 66: 583-590.

Langsjoen PH, Folkers K, Lyson K, Muratsu K, Lyson T. (1990) Pronounced increase of survival of patients with cardiomyopathy when treated with coenzyme Q10 and conventional therapy. *International Journal of Tissue Reactions XIII* (3): 163-168.

Lavie CJ. (1992) Marked benefit with sustained-release niacin (vitamin B3) therapy in patients with isolated very low levels of high-density lipoprotein cholesterol and coronary artery disease. *The American Journal of Cardiology* 69: 1093-1085.

Lawn RM. (1992) Lipoprotein (a) in heart disease. *Scientific American*. June: 54-60.

Lehr HA, Frei B, Arfors KE. (1994) Vitamin C prevents cigarette smoke-induced leucocyte aggregation and adhesion to endothelium in vivo. *Proceedings of the National Academy of Sciences, USA* 91: 7688-7692.

Levine M. (1986) New concepts in the biology and biochemistry of ascorbic acid. *New England Journal of Medicine* 314: 892-902.

Liu VJ, Abernathy RP. (1982) Chromium and insulin in young subjects with normal glucose tolerance. *American Journal of Clinical Nutrition* 25: 661-667.

Maeda N, et. al. (2000) Aortic wall damage in mice unable to synthesize ascorbic acid. *Proceedings of the National Academy of Sciences, USA* 97(2): 841-846.

Mann GV, Newton P. (1975) The membrane transport of ascorbic acid. Second Conference on Vitamin C. *Annals of the New York Academy of Sciences* 258: 243-252.

Mather HM, et. al. (1979) Hypomagnesemia in diabetes. *Clinical and Chemical Acta* 95: 235-242.

McBride PE and Davis JE. (1992) Cholesterol and cost-effectiveness implications for practice, policy, and research. *Circulation* 85: 1939-1941.

McCarron DA, Morris CD, Henry HJ and Stanton JL. (1984) Blood pressure and nutrient intake in the United States. *Science* 224: 1392-1398.

McNair P, et. al. (1978) Hypomagnesemia, a risk factor in diabetic retinopathy. *Diabetes* 27: 1075-1077.

Miccoli R, Marchetti P, Sampietro T, Benzi L, Tognarelli M, Navalesi R. (1984) Effects of pantethine on lipids and apolipoproteins in hypercholesterolemic diabetic and non-diabetic patients. *Current Therapeutic Research* 36: 545-549.

Mikami H, et. al. (1990) Blood pressure response to dietary calcium intervention in humans. *American Journal of Hypertension* 3: 147-151.

Moore TJ. (1995) *Deadly Medicine*. Simon & Schuster, New York.

Newman TB and Hulley SB. (1996) Carcinogenicity of lipid-lowering drugs. *Journal of the American Medical Association* 275: 55-60.

Niendorf A, Rath M, Wolf K, Peters S, Arps H, Beisiegel U, Dietel M. (1990) Morphological detection and quantification of lipoprotein (a) deposition in atheromatous lesions of human aorta and coronary arteries. *Virchow's Archives of Pathological Anatomy* 417: 105-111.

Nunes GL, Sgoutas DS, Redden RA, Sigman SR, Gravanis MB, King SB, Berk BC. (1995) Combination of Vitamin C and E alters the response to coronary balloon injury in the pig. *Arteriosclerosis, Thrombosis and Vascular Biology* 15: 156-165.

Opie LH. (1979) Review: Role of carnitine in fatty acid metabolism of normal and ischemic myocardium. *American Heart Journal* 97: 375-388.

Paolisso G, et. al. (1993) Pharmacologic doses of vitamin E improve insulin action in healthy subjects and in non-insulin-dependent diabetic patients. *American Journal of Clinical Nutrition* 57: 650-656.

Paterson JC. (1941) Some factors in the causation of intimal hemorrhages and in the precipitation of coronary thrombi. *Canadian Medical Association Journal* 44: 114-120.

Pauling L. (1986) *How to Live Longer and Feel Better.* W.H. Freeman and Company, New York.

Pfleger R, Scholl F. (1937) Diabetes und vitamin C. *Wiener Archiv für Innere Medizin* 31: 219-230.

Psaty BM, Heckbert SR, Koepsell TD, et. al. (1995) The risk of myocardial infarction associated with antihypertensive drug therapies. *Journal of the American Medical Association* 274: 620-625.

Rath M, Niendorf A, Reblin T, Dietel M, Krebber HJ, Beisiegel U. (1989) Detection and quantification of lipoprotein (a) in the arterial wall of 107 coronary bypass patients. *Arteriosclerosis* 9: 579-592.

Rath M, Pauling L. (1990a) Hypothesis: Lipoprotein (a) is a surrogate for ascorbate. *Proceedings of the National Academy of Sciences, USA* 87: 6204-6207.

Rath M, Pauling L (1990b) Immunological evidence for the accumulation of lipoprotein (a) in the atherosclerotic lesion of the hypoascorbemic guinea pig. *Proceedings of the National Academy of Sciences, USA* 87: 9388-9390.

Rath M, Pauling L. (1991a) Solution to the puzzle of human cardiovascular disease: Its primary cause is ascorbate deficiency, leading to the deposition of lipoprotein (a) and fibrinogen/fibrin in the vascular wall. *Journal of Orthomolecular Medicine* 6: 125-134.

Rath M, Pauling L. (1991b) Apoprotein(a) is an adhesive protein. *Journal of Orthomolecular Medicine* 6: 139-143.

Rath M, Pauling L. (1992a) A unified theory of human cardiovascular disease leading the way to the abolition of this disease as a cause for human mortality. *Journal of Orthomolecular Medicine* 7: 5-15.

Rath M, Pauling L. (1992b) Plasmin-induced proteolysis and the role of apoprotein(a), lysine, and synthetic lysine analogs. *Journal of Orthomolecular Medicine* 7: 17-23.

Rath M. (1992c) Lipoprotein-a reduction by ascorbate. *Journal of Orthomolecular Medicine* 7: 81-82.

Rath M. (1992d) Solution to the puzzle of human evolution. *Journal of Orthomolecular Medicine* 7: 73-80.

Rath M. (1992e) Reducing the risk for cardiovascular disease with nutritional supplements. *Journal of Orthomolecular Medicine* 7: 153-162.

Rath M. (1993) A new era in medicine. *Journal of Orthomolecular Medicine* 8: 134-135.

Rath M. (1996) The Process of Eradicating Heart Disease Has Become Irreversible. *Journal of Applied Nutrition* 48: 22-33.

Rath M, Niedzwiecki A. (1996) Nutritional Supplement Program Halts Progression of Early Coronary Atherosclerosis Documented by Ultrafast Computed Tomography. *Journal of Applied Nutrition* 48: 68-78.

Rath M, Niedzwiecki A. (1997) Progression of early stages of coronary calcifications can be stopped by the synergistic effect of vitamins and essential nutrients. *Atherosclerosis* 134: 333.

Rhoads GG, Dahlen G, Berg K, Morton NE, Dannenberg AL. (1986) Lp(a) Lipoprotein as a risk factor for myocardial infarction. *Journal of the American Medical Association* 256: 2540-2544.

Riales RR, Albrink MJ. Effect of chromium chloride supplementation on glucose tolerance and serum lipids including high-density lipoprotein of adult men. *American Journal of Clinical Nutrition* 34: 2670-2678.

Riemersma RA, Wood DA, Macintyre CCA, Elton RA, Gey KF, Oliver MF. (1991) Risk of angina pectoris and plasma concentrations of vitamins A, C, and E and carotene. *The Lancet* 337: 1-5.

Rimm EB, Stampfer MJ, Ascherio AA, Giovannucci E, Colditz GA, Willett WC. (1993) Vitamin E consumption and the risk of coronary heart disease in men. *New England Journal of Medicine* 328: 1450-1449.

Rivers JM. (1975) Oral contraceptives and ascorbic acid. *American Journal of Clinical Nutrition* 28: 550-554.

Rizzon P, Biasco G, Di Biase M, Boscia F, Rizzo U, Minafra F, Bortone A, Silprandi N, Procopio A, Bagiella E, Corsi M. (1989) High doses of L-carnitine in acute myocardial infarction: metabolic and antiarrhythmic effects. *European Heart Journal* 10: 502-508.

Robinson K, Arheart K, Refsum H, et. al. (1998) Low circulating folate and vitamin B6 concentrations: risk factors for stroke, peripheral vascular disease, and coronary artery disease. *Circulation* 97(5): 437-43. Erratum in: *Circulation* (1999) 99(7): 983.

Rudolph W. (1939) Vitamin C und Ernährung. Enke Verlag Stuttgart.

Salonen JT, Salonen R, Ihanainen M, Parviainen M, Seppänen R, Seppänen K, Rauramaa R. (1987) Vitamin C deficiency and low linolenate intake associated with elevated blood pressure: The Kuopio Ischemic Heart Disease Risk Factor Study. *Journal of Hypertension* 5 (Supplement 5): S521-S524.

Salonen JT, Salonen R, Seppäneen K, Rinta-Kiikka S, Kuukka M, Korpela H, Alfthan G, Kantola M, Schalch W. (1991) Effects of antioxidant supplementation on platelet function: a randomized pair-matched, placebo-controlled, double-blind trial in men with low antioxidant status. *American Journal of Clinical Nutrition* 53: 1222-1229.

Sauberlich HE, Machlin LJ. (Editors) (1992) Beyond deficiency: New views on the function and health effects of vitamins. *Annals of the New York Academy of Sciences* v. 669.

Shimon I, Almog S, Vered Z, et. al. (1995) Improved left ventricular function after thiamine supplementation in patients with congestive heart failure receiving long-term furosemide therapy. *American Journal of Medicine* 98: 485-90.

315

Smith HA, Jones TC. (1958) *Veterinary Pathology.* Lea and Febiger, Philadelphia.

Sokoloff B, Hori M, Saelhof CC, Wrzolek T, Imai T. (1966) Aging, atherosclerosis and ascorbic acid metabolism. *Journal of the American Gerontology Society* 14: 1239-1260.

Som S, Basu S, Mukherjee D, Deb S, Choudhury PR, Mukherjee S, Chatterjee SN, Chatterjee IB. (1981) Ascorbic acid metabolism in diabetes mellitus. *Metabolism* 30: 572-577.

Spittle CR (1971) Atherosclerosis and Vitamin C. *Lancet* 2: 1280-1.

Stampfer MJ, Hennekens CH, et. al. (1993) Vitamin E consumption and the risk of coronary disease in women. *New England Journal of Medicine* 328(20): 1444-9.

Stankova L, Riddle M, Larned J, Burry K, Menashe D, Hart J, Bigley R. (1984) Plasma ascorbate concentrations and blood cell dehydroascorbate transport in patients with diabetes mellitus. *Metabolism* 33: 347-353.

Stephens NG, Parsons A, Schofield PM, et. al. (1996) Randomized controlled trial of vitamin E in patients with coronary disease: Cambridge Heart Antioxidant Study (CHAOS). *Lancet* 347: 781-6.

Stepp W, Schroeder H, Altenburger E. (1935) Vitamin C und Blutzucker. *Klinische Wochenschrift* 14 [26]: 933-934.

Stryer L. (1988) *Biochemistry. 3rd edition.* W.H. Freeman and Company, New York.

Tarry WC. (1994) L-arginine improves endothelium-dependent vasorelaxation and reduces initial hyperplasia after balloon angioplasty. *Arteriosclerosis and Thrombosis* 14: 938-943.

Teo KK, Salim Y. (1993) Role of magnesium in reducing mortality in acute myocardial infarction: A review of the evidence. *Drugs* 46[3]: 347-359.

Thomsen JH, Shug AL, Yap VU, et. al. (1979) Improved pacing tolerance of the ischemic human myocardium after administration of carnitine. *American Journal of Cardiology* 43: 300-306.

Toufexis A. (1992) The New Scoop on Vitamins. *Time Magazine* April 6: 54-59.

Turlapaty P, Altura BM. (1980) Magnesium deficiency produces spasms of coronary arteries: Relationship to etiology of sudden death ischemic heart disease. *Science* 208: 198-200.

Virchow R. (1859) *Cellular Pathologie.* August Hirschwald, Berlin.

*Vital Statistics of the United States.* US Department of Health and Human Services, National Center for Health Statistics, 1994.

Widman L, et. al. (1993) The dose-dependent reduction in blood pressure through administration of magnesium. A double blind placebo-controlled cross-over study. *American Journal of Hypertension* 6(1): 161-165.

Willis GC, Light AW, Gow WS. (1954) Serial arteriography in atherosclerosis. *Canadian Medical Association Journal* 71: 562-568.

*World Health Statistics.* World Health Organization, Geneva, 1994.

Yokoyama T, Date C, Kokubo Y, et. al. (2000) Serum vitamin C concentration was inversely associated with subsequent 20-year incidence of stroke in a Japanese rural community. The Shibata Study. *Stroke* 31(10): 2287-94.

Zenker G, Koeltringer P, Bone G, Kiederkorn K, Pfeiffer K, Jürgens G. (1986) Lipoprotein (a) as a strong indicator for cardiovascular disease. *Stroke* 17: 942-945.

# Notes

Visit the world's leading website on natural health for the latest information on vitamin research and the Cellular Medicine approach to cardiovascular disease and other health problems:

# www.dr-rath-research.org

Visit the world's leading website about the battle for natural health freedom and learn what you can do to help build a new patient-oriented health care system anywhere in the world:

# www.dr-rath-health-foundation.org

You may also be interested in other books by Dr. Matthias Rath:

- *Cancer*
  The breakthrough in cancer research

- *Ten Years That Changed Medicine Forever*
  The personal record of Dr. Rath's battle for natural health freedom

- *Good Health-Do It Yourself!*
  Documentation of health improvements in patients with the Cellular Medicine approach

**For more information:**

**USA and Canada:**
Dr. Rath Educational Services USA, BV
1260 Memorex Drive, Suite 100
Santa Clara, CA 95050

Tel: 1-800-624-2442
Fax: 1-408-748-1726

**Europe:**
MR Publishing, B.V.
Postbus 859
7600 AW Almelo
The Netherlands
Tel: +31-546 533 333
Fax: +31-546 533 323